Nursing Calculations & IV Therapy

FOR DUMMIES®

A Wiley Brand

by Claire Boyd RGN

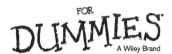

FOR DUMMIES®
A Wiley Brand

Nursing Calculations & IV Therapy For Dummies®

Published by: **John Wiley & Sons, Ltd., The Atrium, Southern Gate, Chichester,** www.wiley.com

This edition first published 2016

© 2016 by John Wiley & Sons, Ltd., Chichester, West Sussex

Registered Office

John Wiley & Sons, Ltd., The Atrium, Southern Gate, Chichester, West Sussex, PO19 8SQ, United Kingdom

For details of our global editorial offices, for customer services and for information about how to apply for permission to reuse the copyright material in this book, please see our website at www.wiley.com.

For general information on our other products and services, please contact our Customer Care Department within the U.S. at 877-762-2974, outside the U.S. at 317-572-3993, or fax 317-572-4002. For technical support, please visit www.wiley.com/techsupport.

Wiley publishes in a variety of print and electronic formats and by print-on-demand. Some material included with standard print versions of this book may not be included in e-books or in print-on-demand. If this book refers to media such as a CD or DVD that is not included in the version you purchased, you may download this material at http://booksupport.wiley.com. For more information about Wiley products, visit www.wiley.com.

A catalogue record for this book is available from the British Library.

ISBN: 978-1-119-11416-1 (pbk); ISBN 978-1-119-11440-6 (ebk); ISBN 978-1-119-11425-3 (ebk)

Printed and bound by CPI Group (UK) Ltd, Croydon, CR0 4YY

C9781119114161_130624

Contents at a Glance

Table of Contents

Introduction

・・

*T*his book is really two for the price of one: a book on – yes, I'm going to use the 'c' word – *calculations* (sends a chill down your spine, doesn't it?) and another book on intravenous (IV) drug administration. As well as offering you great value, this approach is necessary, because you first need to know your maths in order to administer medications.

Don't panic, however! This book takes you by the hand and walks you gently through the basics, before leading you on to the more advanced stuff. I've worked for many years in healthcare and taught thousands of individuals how to work out their drug administration calculations. I've also listened to their concerns about how scary giving IV drugs is, because they fear that they may get something wrong. With their assistance, I've formulated tricks of the trade to help them (and now you) become confident and competent in delivering IV therapy.

This book helps you get to grips with the maths competency side of your nurse training (or similar course, such as assistant practitioner, operating department practitioner and so on). You're required to pass maths tests along the way throughout this training. Also, when you've qualified – or are about to qualify – you need to prove your maths ability by taking an IV calculations test, before being trained to administer IV drugs.

Even then it's not over! After you pass the IV calculations test, you're ready to attend the IV study training: this book also provides you with the skills to perform this clinical skill.

About This Book

Calculations and IV therapy are two huge subjects in their own right, but this book aims to provide you with what you need to know, covering the major areas in an easy-to-read format. True, you may have to read some of the sections more than once to get the point, but don't become disheartened. Keep with it to increase your knowledge and skills.

To be honest, I wish this book had been available when I first started administering IV therapy! I'd have saved a lot of time and effort.

One convention that I do use to help you: I often abbreviate units of measurement into what you see in practice, especially in equations and exercises: for example 'g' for grams, 'mg' for milligrams and 'ml' (you may sometimes see 'mL') for millilitres.

Foolish Assumptions

Rightly or wrongly, I make the following assumptions about you:

- ✔ You're a student nurse, midwife or other practising caregiver.
- ✔ You have a certain standard of mathematical ability from secondary school and a healthcare training facility.
- ✔ You have a general working knowledge of basic nursing skills and an understanding of common medical terminology.
- ✔ You want to help people in your care in a kind and compassionate manner to the best of your ability.

Icons Used in This Book

Throughout the book, you come across icons indicating key ideas and information.

This icon gives you handy hints as suggestions or recommendations. You probably don't want to skip over this material, because the information is sure to be useful.

This icon represents important information you really don't want to miss.

Here I provide practical examples to help get across the necessary point.

This icon informs you of something to be aware of: watch out!

Here you get a chance to try out your newly developed skills.

This icon relays what you can call extra information: interesting and useful, but not essential to know.

Beyond the Book

I provide a Cheat Sheet chock-full with lots of helpful information that you can refer to on a regular basis. The Cheat Sheet is at www.dummies.com/ cheatsheet/nursingcalculationsandivtherapyuk.

The printed book isn't the be-all-and-end-all these days. I've also put together some online bonus bits and pieces (at www.dummies.com/extras/ nursingcalculationsandivtherapyuk) to help you take things further.

Where to Go from Here

You don't have to read *For Dummies* books linearly; you can open this book at any section that takes your fancy. If you're unsure where to begin, do as the song says, 'Start at the very beginning, Doe a deer, a female deer, Ray, a drop of golden sun . . .' In other words, start at Chapter 1, which gives you an overview of the whole book, highlighting the broad concepts I cover in each chapter.

Part I
Getting Started with Nursing Calculations and IV Therapy

getting started
with

nursing
calculations &
IV therapy

In this part . . .

- ✔ Use the practice-makes-perfect theory and check your understanding of working with fractions and decimals.

- ✔ Become familiar with working with percentages, averages and ratios, because these skills are often used in healthcare to give a quick indication of specific quantity and when making comparisons.

- ✔ Know how to use moles, millimoles and solution concentrates in order to describe the amount of substance and for electrolyte measurements: for example, 'body sodium levels 133–146 mmol/l'.

- ✔ Interpret doctors' instructions on prescription charts and medical terminology, including the 24-hour clock, so that when administering medications you know that '0800 hours' means '8:00 a.m.' and '20:00' hours means '8:00 p.m.', to avoid any confusion.

Chapter 1

Getting the Lowdown on Nursing Calculations and IV Therapy

In This Chapter

▶ Understanding the basic maths required for healthcare

▶ Knowing IV therapy and its correct administration

▶ Being clear on complications

*I*ntravenous (IV) therapy is one of the most common clinical skills that healthcare professionals perform. It includes administering IV drugs, fluid replacement (including blood and blood products), *cytotoxic* therapy (chemotherapy) and *parenteral nutrition* (which doesn't mean your mum and dad providing a hot meal when you pop home to get your washing done (!) but feeding 'not via the alimentary canal'). Intravenous therapy can also take the form of administering emergency fluids and medications, such as when individuals have sustained huge blood loss, and/or to convert heart arrhythmias back to sinus rhythm.

In this chapter, I describe how this book takes you through the whole IV process – showing you how to walk before you can run. I help you get to grips with the mathematics and formulae necessary to work out the amounts of drugs or fluids to administer through the main routes, including oral, and translating doctors' written instructions (which can be tricky at the best of times!).

This book also describes the types of IV therapy and how they can relate to patients' blood tests obtained by venepuncture (flip to Chapter 11 for more) as well as their medical condition. I explore methods of getting the medications into the IV route as well as looking at the legal and professional aspects of IV therapy and complications associated with specific routes of administration.

Whatever your reason for entering healthcare, you share a common goal with all nurses and other healthcare professionals. You want to make your sick patients better, keep your healthy patients healthy and provide high-quality care to people, including those at their end-of-life journey.

This aim is encompassed within the culture of 'compassionate care' – known as the 6 Cs:

- ✔ Care
- ✔ Compassion
- ✔ Competence
- ✔ Communication
- ✔ Courage
- ✔ Commitment

Practices can, of course, vary among hospitals and clinical areas. Adhere to your own employer's policies and procedures at all times and document all your actions.

Increasing Your Confidence in Healthcare-Related Maths

The Nursing and Midwifery Council (www.nmc.org.uk) specifically states that to become a registered nurse, you need to be competent in calculations that involve the following: 'tablets and capsules, liquid medicines, injections, intravenous infusions including unit dose, sub- and multiple unit dose, complex calculation and SI conversion' – quite a mouthful, but not as scary as it sounds.

For this reason, nursing students, midwives, assistant practitioners and any healthcare professionals involved in the administration of medicines undergo vigorous calculations testing throughout their training, in order to be able to perform drug calculations accurately.

As a healthcare care professional, when you want to administer IV drugs you attend a study session to discover the requirements of IV therapy. Usually before attending the session, you undertake a higher-level maths test in order to prove your maths competence. Many individuals like to revise a few of the basics, before progressing to the higher-level maths.

The wise saying (by the poet John Donne if you want to impress your friends!) goes that 'no man is an island'. In the healthcare environment, this quote indicates that a patient isn't just a physiological medical condition, but a living, breathing being with many elements (the *biopsychosocial* approach to care). In short, care isn't just about working out the drug dosage to administer to the patient, to relieve the biological element of her needs; care involves treating the patient holistically.

Beginning with the basics

Much of the maths you need to become conversant with in the healthcare setting involve fractions, decimals and percentages.

Fractions

Like contestants on *The Voice,* fractions come in four forms (that's got you thinking, hasn't it!):

- ✔ **Common fractions (also known as vulgar fractions):** For example, 1 tablet needs to be cut into two, equates to 1 tablet ÷ 2 = ½.

- ✔ **Decimal fractions:** For example, when needing 0.45 ml (sometimes appears as mL) from 1 ml of liquid medication, 1 is the whole decimal number and 0.45 is a fraction of this whole number (being less than half).

- ✔ **Percentage fractions:** For example, administering a 1-litre (1,000-ml) bag of 5% glucose equates to 5 parts of glucose per every 100 parts of fluid.

- ✔ **Ratio:** For example, 25 patients are on ward 9B, 10 are being transferred to other wards today, with 5 of the 25 patients being discharged home, equals 25:10:5 or 5:2:1.

Decimals

Decimal numbers are built on the metric system, describing tenths, hundredths and thousandths of a number. For example, 1.25 is equal to one whole unit, plus a fraction of one (25 hundredths).

Some calculations require a conversion from the older imperial system of measurement into the metric system. An example is weighing scales showing stones and pounds instead of kilograms. In such cases, you need to know the conversion factors, such as 1 kilogram = 2.2 pounds. Chapter 8 shows how to conduct these conversions.

Chapter 2 covers the metric units and system and Chapter 3 takes you through your fractions and decimals basics.

Percentages

A percentage is a common way of expressing an amount relating to a whole. In healthcare you need to know information such as how much of a drug is in a solution, such as 0.9% sodium chloride in 1 litre of fluid (Chapter 5 has all the gen on solution concentrates).

You work this amount out as follows: (0.9 ÷ 100) × 1,000 ml = 9 grams. You now know that 9 grams of sodium chloride are in a 1-litre bag of fluid.

Chapter 4 takes you through your percentages calculations, as well as other basics, such as averages and ratios.

Choosing to Use Bundles

Often you're required to work with quite complicated and complex mathematics in order to administer the correct amount of medication to the patient.

One method that can help with this task is the *bundle system* (which is where you break down the numbers into smaller units).

Imagine that 10 milligrams of a drug is presented as 5 millilitres. The patient is prescribed 2.5 milligrams of the drug and you need to find out how much this amount equates to in millilitres. You do so simply by breaking down the dose into smaller units:

- 10 mg = 5 ml
- 5 mg = 2.5 ml
- 2.5 mg = 1.25 ml

Therefore, the patient requires 1.25 millilitres of the drug.

(By the way, this example is also an example of the useful examples I provide throughout this book – as examples!)

Working out the tablet/capsule drug dosages

When a patient is prescribed, say, 300 milligrams of a medication presented as 300 milligrams per tablet, you know to administer one tablet. Simple. Sometimes, however, the maths can get a little more complicated, which is where the formula method or approach comes in useful.

Here's one useful formula that you encounter throughout this book:

What you want ÷ what you've got

In other words, the prescribed amount divided by how the drug is presented in its packaging.

A patient requires 45 milligrams (that's what you want) of a drug presented as 135 milligrams per tablet (that's what you've got). Therefore, you use the above formula:

45 ÷ 135 = 0.33 mg, which equates to one third of the tablet

You can reverse-check this answer by multiplying 45 by 3 = 135 milligrams.

Chapter 8 takes you through the safety precautions of administering medications, because you'd never break a tablet into a third – the resulting tablet part may not be an accurate third. Plus, Chapter 9 discusses the process by which pills work in the body when taken orally.

Calculating liquid drug dosages

Liquid medications, including those required for injection (see Chapter 10), are presented in liquid format (or need to be reconstituted in liquid). You measure them into a pot, oral syringe or injectable syringe, using the same formula as for tablets and capsules (see the preceding section), but you have to add the extra aspect of 'volume'. So the formula becomes:

(What you want ÷ What you've got) × Volume

For a prescribed dose of 250 milligrams of amoxicillin, from an ampoule containing 125 milligrams in 5 millilitres, you add the numbers into this formula:

(250 mg ÷ 125 mg) × 5 ml = 10 ml

In order to work out these drug dosages, good practice is to get someone to check your answer independently where possible and to use a calculator for the more complex calculations.

Chapter 8 goes through the common oral and injectable formulae for working out drug dosages, and Chapter 12 looks at the more advanced ones.

Monitoring Your Patients

As a healthcare professional, you need to measure and record details of your patients' conditions. This information relates to their vital signs, prescriptions, fluid levels and any indications of deterioration. You need to know the important methods and documents for recording these details inside out.

Visiting the realm of vital signs: Physiological measurements

When a patient's respiratory rate and heart rate rise, you need to investigate the reason why and provide an appropriate treatment. For example, you may need to administer analgesics and/or anti-emetics if the patient is in pain or feeling sick. In other words, you need to apply nursing calculations in all aspects of the patient's care, not just when administering medications. The *physiological measurements* – or vital signs (see Chapter 7) – are often abbreviated to TPR and BP (meaning temperature, pulse and respirations and blood pressure).

When administering medications to patients, you need to look at the whole picture and understand that the prescription chart isn't something to follow blindly. For example, you don't administer anti-hypertensive medication to a patient who's hypotensive, or give a drug when you've just found out that the patient previously suffered an allergic reaction to it (for details about adverse reactions, check out Chapter 13). You use your noggin (brain) to work out that you need to discuss this issue with the doctor.

Interpreting the prescription chart

Before administering medications, you need to be familiar with the abbreviations on the prescription chart. In the community (anything out of the hospital setting), this chart is often called the *Medication Administration Records and Requests* document (or MARRs sheet).

Whatever the specific document you use, understanding the instructions is vital.

Another factor when reading the prescription chart is whether the medication has been prescribed using the correct _non-proprietary_ name (that is, the chemical or generic name) or the _proprietary_ name (the brand or trade name). To avoid confusion, drugs should be prescribed using the approved generic name. For example, salbutamol (albuterol) is the drug's non-proprietary name, whereas its proprietary name is Ventolin.

Generally speaking, don't use too many abbreviations, apart from the approved ones, because different clinical areas sometimes use different abbreviations. For example, DOA can mean 'dead on arrival' in an emergency unit but 'date of admission' in a ward unit. Unsurprisingly, patients object to being declared dead when they've just arrived for a 15-minute cataract procedure!

Chapter 6 looks at interpreting instructions.

Finding out about the fluid chart

The _fluid chart_ is an important document, which when completed correctly establishes the patient's fluid balance. The _fluid balance_ (see Chapter 7) relates to the difference between the amount of fluid taken into the body and the amount excreted or lost.

Accurately monitoring a patient's fluid balance is crucial to a patient's well-being, because the body works within narrow parameters and is always striving for _homeostasis_ (balance). In other words, any water loss needs to be replaced in order for the body's water volume to remain constant.

Completing a fluid chart is simply about recording the amount of all drinks, IV fluids and so on going into the patient's body. You then add up all the fluid that has left the body, taking this amount away from the input amount. The result is the fluid balance.

When the intake is greater than the output amount, a _positive balance_ is recorded, but if the intake amount is less than output the fluid balance is recorded as _negative_. The balance is usually viewed over a couple of days, because sometimes the body is playing 'catch-up'.

Sometimes, when you're rushed off your feet, you can tally up these figures inaccurately. As a result, the patient may be prescribed more or less fluids wrongly, which can have an adverse effect on the person's well-being.

Reading the NEWS chart

Many healthcare settings use the National Early Warning Score (NEWS) observation chart as a 'surveillance' system to identify and monitor patients deteriorating. The reason is simple: picking up these signs saves lives.

Research shows that 80 per cent of NHS patients across the UK experiencing a cardiac arrest had physiological abnormalities present 12–24 hours prior to the cardiac arrest.

The NEWS charts are colour-coded in order to demonstrate the severity of the patient's condition – a high NEWS score indicates a severe illness. No point knowing how many pills to give your sick patient if you don't observe the poor soul deteriorating! Chapter 7 shows you how to use these charts.

Administering IV Therapy

Intravenous therapy is medics' chosen route when they need to deliver fluids and medications as quickly as possible to the patient. IV therapy is also used in order to give substances that can't be administered by any other route. For example, unless you're a vampire, a blood transfusion is administered via the IV route as opposed to the oral route (sink your teeth into Chapter 17 for more details).

Getting under the skin of the IV route

Doctors use a variety of methods of administering drugs via the IV route. The most common types of IV administration include the following:

- ✔ **Peripheral IVs:** The tip of these devices sits in the vein, usually in the hand or arm. These short-term devices are used to deliver IV drugs or fluids (flip to Chapter 16 for details).

- ✔ **IV bolus push:** When a specific dose of a medication is given via a bolus through a peripheral or central device (see Chapter 15).

- ✔ **Central lines:** These devices are placed in the chest, neck, groin, leg, arm or scalp. The catheter is sited in the veins of the central venous system, such as the superior vena cava or inferior vena cava (Chapter 16 has all about central lines).

- ✔ **Infusion pumps, syringe drivers and patient controlled analgesia (PCA) pumps:** These electronic devices are set to infuse fluids or medications via an automatic pump intermittently or continuously. Syringe drivers generally administer smaller controlled doses of medication over a prescribed duration. PCAs give patients control over their analgesic administration, because they can self-administer their medication. (Check out Chapter 14 for more on these devices.)

- ✔ **Volumetric pumps:** These devices administer medications such as sodium chloride 0.9% via an administration set to a peripheral device sited in, for example, the patient's arm. Depending on the infusate, the administration set delivers 20 drops per millilitre for clear fluids and 15 drops per millilitre for blood and thickened fluids. A microdrip system infuses smaller amounts of fluids per hour. (Pop to Chapter 14 for more on volumetric pumps.)

- ✔ **Continuous and intermittent infusions:** Continuous infusions deliver medications or fluids at a constant rate, whereas intermittent infusions deliver medications or fluids at specific times and at designated intervals (see Chapter 15).

Appreciating the advantages of IV administration

The IV route has many advantages over other routes of drug administration. You can:

- ✔ Achieve a rapid response of the medication if a patient is having a cardiac arrest

- ✔ Provide a constant therapeutic effect, such as via continuous infusion

- ✔ Still give medication if the patient is nil by mouth (NBM)

- ✔ Still administer the medication if the patient is unable to undergo an intramuscular injection, due to being a haemophiliac

- ✔ Give medications that may not be absorbed via the oral route

- ✔ Administer medication to unconscious patients

- ✔ Correct fluids and electrolyte imbalances promptly

Looking Out for the Complications of IV Therapy

Make no mistake about it, despite all the advantages of IV therapy that I lay out in the preceding section, the process isn't without its complications. Here are some potential complications that you may face and how to deal with them.

Understanding the disadvantages of IV administration

The IV route has the following disadvantages as a means of fluid and drug administration:

- ✔ Side effects to the drug usually more immediate and severe
- ✔ Risk of embolism
- ✔ Risk of microbial contamination/infection
- ✔ Risk of infiltration
- ✔ Risk of extravasation
- ✔ Risk of phlebitis
- ✔ Increased risk of fluid overload
- ✔ Risk of speed shock
- ✔ Problems with compatibility/stability of medicines

Chapters 18 and 19 give more information around these topics.

Preventing infection

One of the major risks of using the IV route is, of course, infection. Hand-washing with liquid soap and water is the single most important means of preventing the spread of infection. Washing with liquid soap and water is often referred as the gold standard of infection control.

Using the *aseptic non-touch technique* (ANTT) is the evidence-based method of administering IV medications. It ensures that asepsis is achieved on the key parts of the equipment that come into direct or indirect contact with the liquid infusion during preparation and administration of the medication.

When preparing medications for patients, the healthcare professional identifies all the key parts and then protects them at all times using the non-touch technique.

Here's the ten-step overview of the ANTT in relation to IV therapy:

1. **Gather together all the equipment.**
2. **Clean the *aseptic field* – the area you working from (injection tray and so on).**
3. **Clean your hands and put on an apron and non-sterile gloves.**
4. **Prepare the medicines and equipment, protecting key parts at all times using the non-touch technique.**
5. **Go to the patient and prepare the access device, after gaining the patient's consent.**
6. **Administer medicines – protecting key parts at all times.**
7. **Dispose of any sharps immediately.**
8. **Remove gloves and apron.**
9. **Wash hands.**
10. **Document your actions.**

Chapter 18 looks at the infection control aspects of IV therapy.

Dealing with pain on IV injection

Before administering IV medications through a peripheral line, you need to undertake an inspection of the site.

If the patient doesn't complain of pain during the cannula *flush* (which isn't a hand at poker, but when you clean out the line – see Chapter 14), but does so on the administration of the drug, this pain may be due to the following reasons:

- ✔ **Hypertonicity:** Where medicines have a higher osmolarity than plasma, which can cause fluids to pass out of blood cells, resulting in cell *lysis* (breaking down of the cell).
- ✔ **Rapid administration:** Inappropriate rapid infusion or insufficient dilution of irritant medications can cause damage to the blood vessels, resulting in pain.

Here's a list of drugs that are known to cause pain on injection:

✔ Dextrose solutions above 10 per cent dilutions

✔ Erythromycin

✔ Phenytoin

✔ Potassium infusions

✔ Sodium bicarbonate 8.4 per cent

✔ Tetracycline

✔ Vancomycin

Chapter 16 looks at access devices and pain. For more on pain management in general and morphine in particular, move gingerly to Chapter 20.

Chapter 2

It's about Units, Innit! The Metric System of Measurement

*W*hen using maths in healthcare, you need a good understanding of the basic principles of the metric system of measurement. Sometimes you're required to work with small units of the whole (the difference between administering a thousandth and a tenth of a unit of medicine can be, quite literally, fatal).

For example, if you take the gram (g) unit of measurement as the whole, but require one-thousandth ($\frac{1}{1,000}$) of this unit, you have the *milli*gram (mg). The 'milli' part is known as a *prefix* in the metric system; prefixes are used to denote multiples and sub-multiples of its units.

In this chapter, I walk you through all the important parts of the metric system as it relates to healthcare, including working with decimals and converting from one unit to another.

Anyone for Tens? Using the Metric System of Measurement

The metric system is an internationally recognised decimal system of measurement. You may also hear people refer to the decimal numeral system as *the base ten system* (or *denary*) due to it having the number 10 as its base.

The decimal system's main features include a standard set of inter-related base units and a standard set of prefixes in the power of 10. In other words, decimals describe 'tenths' of a number, meaning in terms of 10.

Table 2-1 shows you that the *base unit* is the number 1. Anything increasing from it is a whole number. Anything decreasing from the base unit of 1 has a zero in front and is therefore part of a number (known as a *fraction*).

Table 2-1	Prefixes from the Base Unit 1	
Prefix	*Abbreviation*	*Multiple/decimal fraction*
Giga	G	1,000,000,000
Mega	M	1,000,000
Kilo	k	1,000
Hecto	h	100
Deca	da	10
BASE UNIT		1
Deci	d	0.1
Centi	c	0.01
Milli	m	0.001
Micro	mcg* or μ	0.000,001
Nano	n	0.000,000,001
Pico	p	0.000,000,000,001
Femto	f	0.000,000,000,000,001

Don't abbreviate 'micro' in healthcare settings, because it can be confused with 'milli'.

The main prefixes that you come into contact with in the healthcare setting are mega, kilo, milli, micro and nano. Micrometres and nanometres are used to measure particularly small anatomical structures, such as blood vessels and cells.

In this section, I help you get to know how to work with decimals in various ways and introduce you to SI units.

Defining SI units

The SI unit stands for *International System of Units* or *(Systeme Internationale)*. This unit is really just another name for the metric system of measurement, being the internationally recognised standard metric system.

Measuring the distance from Europe

A version of the metric system of measurement has been around for centuries – it was first used in France in 1799 (something else you can blame the French for!). This system is now generally accepted in most countries.

The United Kingdom NHS adopted the SI system in 1975, for use in medical practice and pharmacy, so that – as the saying goes – everyone is 'singing from the same song sheet'. Unfortunately, just to confuse matters, the imperial system of measurement is also still in everyday legal use in the UK: this system includes inches, feet, miles and yards; acres; fluid ounces, pints, quart and gallons; grains, ounces, pounds and stones. Phew! (The SI system doesn't look quite so daunting now, does it? Perhaps you should thank the French after all!)

This situation does mean that you may sometimes need to change imperial measures into the metric system, because a patient only knows his weight in pounds and ounces and height in feet and inches. In Chapter 8 you can find conversion tables to help do the work for you!

For some background, see the nearby sidebar 'Measuring the distance from Europe'.

The main SI units you need to use in healthcare – called *SI Base Units* – are those used to measure the following (check out Table 2-2 for more):

- **Weight:** Kilogram (kg).
- **Volume:** Litre (l or L).
- **Amount of substance:** Mole (mol – check out Chapter 5).
- **Length:** Metre (m).
- **Temperature:** Kelvin (K). A temperature scale (SI units) from which temperatures after 'absolute zero' don't exist. Most people probably think of metric temperatures as being in Celsius/Centigrade (such as body temperature).

Table 2-2   Metric Weight, Volume, Length and Substance Equivalences and Abbreviations

	Abbreviation	Equivalent	Abbreviation
Equivalences of weight			
1 kilogram	kg	1,000 grams	g
1 gram	g	1,000 milligrams	mg
1 milligram	mg	1,000 micrograms	mcg* or μ

(continued)

Table 2-2 *(continued)*

	Abbreviation	*Equivalent*	*Abbreviation*
1 microgram	mcg* or μ	1,000 nanograms	ng*
1 nanogram	ng*	1,000 picograms	pg*
Equivalences of volume			
1 litre	l or L	1,000 millilitres	ml or mL
1 millilitre	ml or mL	1,000 microlitres	mcg* or μL
Equivalences of length			
1 kilometre	km	1,000 metres	m
1 metre	m	1,000 kilometres	km
Equivalences of amount of substance			
1 mole	mol	1,000 millimoles	mmol
1 millimole	mmol	1,000 micromoles	mcmol*

*Don't use these abbreviations on prescription charts and similar, because of the risk of misreading.

The litre isn't formally part of the SI but has become accepted as an International System of Unit.

From Table 2-2, you can see that 1 litre is the same as 1,000 ml. So, if you need to give half a litre, you may see this expressed as 0.5 litres or as 500 ml (because half of 1,000 ml is 500).

People shouldn't employ abbreviations when using micrograms, nanograms, picograms, micromoles or microlitres in the healthcare setting on prescription charts, in case they get mistaken for another unit (such as mcg for mg). You know that medics don't always write with the most legible handwriting!

To help you become familiar with SI units, here are some more equivalent examples of weight, volume and amount of substance:

Original weight	*Equivalent weight*
0.4 g	400 mg
500 mg	0.5 g
2 mcg	2,000 ng

A nanogram is equal to one billionth of a gram = 0.000,000,001 grams.

Original volume	*Equivalent volume*
0.1 L	100 ml
750 ml	0.7 l

Original amount of substance	Equivalent amount of substance
0.25 mol	250 mmol
750 mmol	0.75 mol

Introducing the decimal unit

A decimal number is a number that's expressed in the counting system that uses units of tens, and it generally means a number that includes a decimal point. This decimal point, or dot, divides the whole number, which is to the left of it, with parts less than a whole number on the right of it. This decimal point goes between the units and tenths.

Numbers to the left of the decimal point are greater than one. Numbers to the right of the decimal point are less than one.

The number 22.3 has 2 tens, 2 units and 3 tenths = $20 + 2 + \frac{3}{10}$.

So, to the right of the decimal point are the tenths, hundredths, thousandths and so on: called the *place value* in decimals.

To try this process for yourself, consider the number 0.954: you know that these figures mean 9 tenths, 5 hundredths and 4 thousandths. To see the number expressed in a visual form, see Figure 2-1.

Figure 2-1:
Visual representation of 0.954.

Millions	Hundred thousands	Ten Thousands	Thousands	Hundreds	Tens	Ones	Decimal point	Tenths	Hundredths	Thousandths	Ten-thousandths	Hundred-thousandths	Millionths
						0		9	5	4			

© John Wiley & Sons, Inc.

So, you know that the number 0.954 isn't a whole number, but part of the number 1. When you've written a number with a decimal point, most of the zeros at the end of the answer become unnecessary:

- 0.2000 becomes 0.2
- 4.00 becomes 4.0
- 7.900 becomes 7.9
- 2.500 becomes 2.5
- 325.000 becomes 325.0

Any number(s) after the decimal dot is known as *the decimal place.* Here are a few more examples of decimal places:

- ✔ 2.76 = two decimal places
- ✔ 35.7 = one decimal place
- ✔ 23.505 = three decimal places
- ✔ 1.42 = two decimal places
- ✔ 19.5000 = four decimal places
- ✔ 6.5 = one decimal place
- ✔ 1.672 = three decimal places

Multiplying decimals

You need to multiply decimals in all sorts of healthcare situations. For example, when working out the dose of a medicine required by a child, you can use the following formula:

Weight (kg) × Dose

If the child is small, you may only have his weight in grams; to use this formula, you need to convert the weight into kilograms (Chapter 3 has loads more on reducing doses for children).

You multiply decimals in the same way as whole numbers, but you do have to take account of the decimal point.

Moving the point to the left

To multiply a decimal, you simply move the decimal point the same number of places to the left as numbers after the decimal point.

Imagine that you want to work out 6.7 × 0.4:

1. **Forget about the decimal point.**

   For instance, you already know that 67 × 4 = 268.

2. **Count the numbers after the decimal point.**

   In this case, 6.7 and 0.4 each have one decimal place and so you need to use two decimal places.

3. **Bounce the decimal point the required number of times to the left.**

   Therefore 268.0 becomes 2.68.

Similarly, $0.67 \times 4 = 2.68$ (two decimal places + no decimal places = two decimal places).

Along the same lines, $6.7 \times 0.04 = 0.268$ (one decimal place + two decimal places = three decimal places).

Of course, as with working out any maths, using a calculator is probably quicker and easier. But like all machinery, calculators can make mistakes – which is why knowing how to work things out for yourself is always best.

Here are some more examples of multiplying decimal numbers:

- $6 \times 6 = 36$
    - $0.6 \times 0.6 = 0.36$ (two decimal places)
    - $0.06 \times 0.06 = 0.0036$ (four decimal places)
    - $0.6 \times 0.006 = 0.0036$ (four decimal places)
- $64 \times 12 = 768$
    - $6.4 \times 0.12 = 0.768$ (three decimal places)
    - $0.64 \times 0.12 = 0.0768$ (four decimal places)
    - $0.064 \times 1.2 = 0.0768$ (four decimal places)
- $6 \times 6 = 36$
    - $0.6 \times 0.06 = 0.036$ (three decimal places)
    - $0.06 \times 0.06 = 0.0036$ (four decimal places)

Moving the point to the right

To multiply a decimal by multiples of 10, 100, 1,000 or 10,000, you simply move the decimal point the same number of places to the right as the number of zeros in the number you're multiplying:

- **To multiply by 10:** Move the decimal point 1 place to the right.
- **To multiply by 100:** Move the decimal point 2 places to the right.
- **To multiply by 1,000:** Move the decimal point 3 places to the right.

So, to multiply $987 \times 1,000$, you count the number of zeros in 1,000 (3) and move the decimal point three places to the right of the number you're multiplying by:

$987 \times 1,000 = 987,000$

Check out these examples of decimals in multiples of 10, 100 and 1,000 being multiplied:

- ✔ $600.0 \times 1,000 = 600,000$ (moving decimal point 3 places to the right)
- ✔ $0.8 \times 10 = 8$ (moving decimal 1 place to the right, because you have only 1 zero in 10)
- ✔ $21.9 \times 100 = 2,190$ (moving decimal point 2 places to the right)
- ✔ $50.0 \times 1,000 = 50,000$ (moving decimal 3 places to the right)
- ✔ $61.35 \times 10 = 613.5$ (moving decimal point 1 place to the right)
- ✔ $2.389 \times 100 = 238.9$ (moving decimal point 2 places to the right)

Dividing decimals

To divide decimals, you use the same process as dividing whole numbers, remembering of course to take the decimal point into account:

- ✔ **To divide by 10:** Move the decimal point 1 place to the left.
- ✔ **To divide by 100:** Move the decimal point 2 places to the left.
- ✔ **To divide by 1,000:** Move the decimal point 3 places to the left.

One method of tackling dividing decimals is initially to ignore the decimal point and put it back in afterwards. So, to calculate $9.15 \div 5$, you proceed as follows:

1. **Work out that 5 goes into 9 once, with 4 left over.**
2. **Calculate that 5 goes into 41 (the leftover 4 and the second digit, the 1) 8 times, with 1 left over.**
3. **5 goes into 15 (the leftover 1 and the last digit, the 5) 3 times.**
4. **Put the decimal point back after the first whole number to give you the answer: 1.83.**

Alternatively, you can choose to put the decimal point in from the start. You get the same answer, 1.83 (that's a relief!).

Here's how to calculate $30.0 \div 12$:

1. **Work out that 12 goes into 30 twice, with 6 left over.**
2. **Calculate that 12 goes into 60 (the leftover 6 and the second digit, the 0) 5 times.**
3. **Put the decimal point back after the first whole number to give you the answer: 2.5.**

To divide a decimal by multiples of 10, 100, 1,000 or 10,000, you simply move the decimal point the same number of places to the left as zeros in the number you're dividing.

To divide 987 ÷ 1,000:

The three zeros in 1,000 means that the decimal point moves three places to the left of the number by which you're dividing:

$$987.0 \div 1,000 = 0.987$$

See how you get on with these questions dividing tens, hundreds and thousands, moving the decimal to the left:

1. $600.0 \div 1,000$
2. $0.8 \div 10$
3. $21.9 \div 100$
4. $50.0 \div 1,000$
5. $61.35 \div 10$
6. $2.389 \div 100$

Here are the answers:

1. $600.0 \div 1,000 = 0.6$ (moving decimal point 3 places to the left)
2. $0.8 \div 10 = 0.08$ (moving decimal point 1 place to the left)
3. $21.9 \div 100 = 0.219$ (moving decimal point 2 places to the left)
4. $50.0 \div 1,000 = 0.05$ (moving decimal point 3 places to the left)
5. $61.35 \div 10 = 6.135$ (moving decimal point 1 place to the left)
6. $2.389 \div 100 = 0.02389$ (moving decimal point 2 places to the left)

Mastering Conversions

In healthcare, you're often asked to administer a medication in milligrams that's presented to you in the gram format. Therefore, you need to remember the basic principles of conversion that I describe in this section.

Imagine that a doctor prescribes the penicillin Flucloxacillin for a patient with a chest infection. The drug is presented as 500 milligrams, but the doctor prescribes '0.25 grams every 6 hours, at least 30 minutes before food'. You can seriously harm your patients if you can't convert grams into milligrams – in this case 0.25 grams into 250 milligrams.

Memorise the following weight and volume conversions:

✔ **Weight:**

- 1 kilogram (kg) = 1,000 grams (g)

- 1 gram (g) = 1,000 milligrams (mg)

- 1 milligram (mg) = 1,000 micrograms (mcg)

- 1 microgram (mcg) = 1,000 nanograms (ng)

- 1 nanogram (ng) = 1,000 picograms (pg)

Don't use abbreviations for units smaller that a milligram (that is, mcg, ng or pg) in the healthcare setting on prescription charts.

✔ **Volume:**

- 1 litre (l) = 1,000 millitres (ml)

This information really comes into its own when you administer medications.

Changing larger units into smaller units

In everyday healthcare, you're often asked to convert one decimal unit into another unit: for example, to change micrograms into milligrams.

This task is simply a matter of knowing that to convert a larger unit to a smaller unit, you multiply by 1,000:

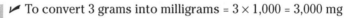

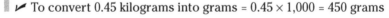

✔ To convert 3 grams into milligrams = 3 × 1,000 = 3,000 mg

✔ To convert 0.45 kilograms into grams = 0.45 × 1,000 = 450 grams

You can also do this task another way, simply by 'bouncing' the decimal point. To multiply by 1,000, you move the decimal point three places to the right.

Therefore, to change 3 grams into milligrams, you move the decimal point three times to the right (× 1,000):

1. **Move it once to the right:** 30.00

2. **Move it a second time to the right:** 300.0

3. **Move it a third time to the right:** 3,000 milligrams

To change 0.45 kilograms into grams, you move the decimal point three times to the right ($\times$ 1,000):

1. **Move it once to the right:** 4.5

2. **Move it a second time to the right:** 45.0

3. **Move it a third time to the right:** 450 grams

Questions

Sit down with a cup of tea or your favourite beverage, and see whether you can change these units into the next smaller unit.

Although I use them for convenience here, don't use the abbreviations for micrograms, nanograms, picograms or microlitres in the healthcare setting, such as on prescription charts: they can get mistaken for another unit (such as mcg for mg).

1. Change 0.72 g into milligrams.

2. Change 1.4 mg into micrograms.

3. Change 0.03 g into milligrams.

4. Change 2.5 l into millilitres.

5. Change 0.7 mg into micrograms.

6. Change 61.25 l into millilitres.

7. Change 2.386 kg into grams.

8. Change 80 kg into grams.

9. Change 0.8 mg to micrograms.

10. Change 1,000 ng into picograms.

Answers

Here are the answers (I hope you didn't peek first!):

1. Changing 0.72 g into milligrams = 720 mg

2. Changing 1.4 mg into micrograms = 1,400 mcg

3. Changing 0.03 g into milligrams = 30 mg

4. Changing 2.5 l into millilitres = 2,500 ml

5. Changing 0.7 mg into micrograms = 700 mg

6. Changing 61.25 l into millilitres = 61,250 ml

7. Changing 2.386 kg into grams = 2,386 g

8. Changing 80 kg into grams = 80,000 g

9. Changing 0.8 mg to micrograms = 800 mcg

10. Changing 1,000 ng into picograms = 1,000,000 pg

Converting smaller units into larger units

Just as you may need to convert one decimal unit into another in order to change larger units into smaller units, you may be required to change smaller units into larger units.

To do this calculation, you simply need to know that to convert a smaller unit to the next larger unit, you divide by 1,000.

You convert 5,500 grams into kilograms as follows: 5,500 ÷ 1,000 = 5.5 kilograms.

Here's how to convert 315 mg to grams: 315 ÷ 1,000 = 0.315 grams.

If you want to use the decimal point 'bounce' method, to divide by 1,000 you move the decimal point three places to the left.

So to change 5,500 mg into grams, you move the decimal place three times to the left (÷ 1,000):

1. Move it once to the left: 550.0

2. Move it a second time to the left: 55.0

3. Move it a third time to the left: 5.5 grams

To change 315 mg into grams, you move the decimal place three times to the left (÷ 1000):

1. Move it once to the left: 31.5

2. Move it a second time to the left: 3.15

3. Move it a third time to the left: 0.315 grams

Questions
Here's your chance to get your hands dirty (well, your brain actually). Change the following units into the next larger unit:

1. 6,000 mg into grams

2. 4,000 ml into litres

   3. 350 ml into litres

   4. 0.7 mcg into milligrams

   5. 4,000 g into kilograms

   6. 10 pg into nanograms

   7. 20 mcg into milligrams

   8. 1,500 mcg into milligrams

   9. 64.5 mcg into milligrams

   10. 50 ml into litres

Answers

   1. 6,000 mg into grams = 6 g

   2. 4,000 ml into litres = 4 l

   3. 350 ml into litres = 0.35 l

   4. 0.7 mcg into milligrams = 0.0007 mg

   5. 4,000 g into kilograms = 4 kg

   6. 10 pg into nanograms = 0.01 ng

   7. 20 mcg into milligrams = 0.02 mg

   8. 1,500 mcg into milligrams = 1.5 mg

   9. 64.5 mcg into milligrams = 0.0645 mg

   10. 50 ml into litres = 0.05 l

Questions

Have a go at changing some more units into the next larger unit:

   1. 6,000 mg

   2. 60 ml

   3. 5,000 ml

   4. 200 mcg

   5. 10 mcg

   6. 7,000 g

   7. 375 g

   8. 185 mcg

   9. 90 mcg

   10. 160 mg

Answers

Here's what you should have written down:

1. 6,000 mg = 6 g
2. 60 ml = 0.06 l
3. 5,000 ml = 5 l
4. 200 mcg = 0.2 mg
5. 10 mcg = 0.01 mg
6. 7,000 g = 7 kg
7. 375 g = 0.375 kg
8. 185 mcg = 0.185 mg
9. 90 mcg = 0.09 mg
10. 160 mg = 0.16 g

Chapter 3

Making a Point: Fractions and Decimals

In This Chapter

▶ Becoming familiar with fractions

▶ Converting between fractions, decimal and percentages

*I*n this chapter you get to tuck into fractions (yum!). Unfortunately, I can't discuss this subject with examples of cutting cherry pies or cakes into parts as you may have done at school – this is a medical book after all, and so you get pills and tablets! Besides, like everyone else, you need to reduce your sugar intake!

In the healthcare setting, many of the medications you receive from the pharmacy are presented in a format to suit adult patients. But children usually require much smaller dosages of the same medication and so you have to be able to calculate the correct amount of the drug to give to them.

To do so, you need to become skilled at working out fractions and decimals, perhaps taking a part or a fraction of the standard dose, or part of a whole number in the case of decimals. Also, knowing how to multiply and divide them allows you to convert from a fraction to a decimal and vice versa. So now that you know the rationale for this chapter and its contents, I'll get on with it!

Getting to Grips with Fractions

A *fraction* is a portion of a whole that indicates division into equal parts. For example, if you divide the number 1 by 2, the answer is a half, expressed as the fraction ½.

So cutting a whole tablet in half gives you 2 halves: 1 large tablet ÷ 2 = ½.

If you need to cut the tablet into four parts, the fraction is ¼: 1 large tablet ÷ 4 = ¼.

Never cut tablets into quarters, because the dosage would be inaccurate. As a rule, tablets should only be cut into half, and then only if they're scored with a line for easy breakage: certainly don't break coated tablets (see Chapter 9). For accuracy, use a tablet cutter to cut scored tablets in half.

In this section you get to work with fractions in all sorts of ways, helping you to administer less than one whole tablet or less than 1 millilitre for injection: in short, part of or a fraction of the whole.

Defining fractions

Many healthcare reports and surveys use fractions to describe investigation findings – for example, comparisons of ethnic groups and babies born prior to full term. You need to question the data – look at the fractions – and see whether they add up (make a whole number).

A fraction is part of a whole number or a number that can be divided by another number. So with the fraction ⅗, you're really saying that 5 is the whole and you have three parts of the 5.

The top and bottom numbers have different names to indicate what they do:

- **Numerator:** The top number of a fraction. The numerator tells you the number of parts of the whole number that are being used: in the case of ⅗, three.

- **Denominator:** The bottom number of a fraction (and not to be confused with Arnold Schwarzenegger's Terminator). The denominator tells you the number of parts into which the whole is divided: in the case of ⅗, five.

When a number is divided by *a factor,* it just means that the answer is a whole number, with nothing left over or remaining. For example, 2 is a factor of 10 because you can divide 2 into 10 five equal times.

For example, if you split a tablet into five equal parts and give three parts to one patient and two parts to another patient (which you'd never do in practice), you can see that 3 + 2 makes the whole tablet with nothing left over.

Simplifying fractions

Sometimes in healthcare you have to know how to simplify fractions, perhaps for working out liquid medications or with parts of equipment.

Here's an unlikely example, purely for illustrative purposes. Imagine that the nurse in charge asks you to use only half of a bandage on the patient's injured hand. But just as you're about to start, another nurse tells you only to use $\frac{3}{6}$ of the roll of bandage. Do you panic? No, because you know that these fractions are the same – $\frac{3}{6}$ can be simplified as ½.

To *simplify* (or *cancel down*) a fraction, you need to divide the numerator and the denominator by the same number, which is called the *common factor* (the opposite of a posh one!). Here's what I mean:

$$\frac{25}{45} = \frac{5}{9}$$

The common factor is 5, because 5 divides into 25 five times, and into 45 nine times, resulting in the fraction $\frac{5}{9}$. So, to reduce a fraction, you need to choose a number that's going to divide exactly into the numerator (top number) and the denominator (bottom number), if such a number exists: if not, the fraction remains as it is – in this case $\frac{5}{9}$. You can see why this process of simplifying fractions is known as *cancellation*.

Try simplifying this fraction yourself: $\frac{100}{225}$

The common factor for both these numbers is 25, which goes into 100 four times and into 225 nine times. Therefore, the cancelled down fraction is $\frac{4}{9}$.

A dehydrated patient has drunk 36 millilitres from a cup of water, which when full contained 48 millilitres; the doctor asks you what fraction of water has been drunk? You need to simplify this fraction $\frac{36}{48} = \frac{18}{24} = \frac{9}{12} = \frac{3}{4}$.

I break the process down into three steps:

1. **Divide 36 (numerator) and 48 (denominator) by the common factor 2.**

   Doing so gives you $\frac{18}{24}$.

2. **Divide 18 and 24 by 2.**

   This gives you $\frac{9}{12}$.

3. **Divide 9 and 12 by 3.**

   You're left with ¾.

Another, quicker approach is to divide the numerator of 36 and the denominator of 48 into 12 to get the same answer in one step.

Adding and subtracting fractions

In healthcare, you sometimes have to add or subtract fractions, perhaps when calculating drug doses or when communicating with members of the multi-disciplinary team such as the dietician. For example, say that Mrs Peters achieved ¾ of her total calorific intake yesterday and only ¼ of it the day before. At the end of the week, you need to tally these up on Mrs Peters' nutrition chart as well as her calorie amount.

Totting up fractions

You use three simple steps to add fractions. Imagine that you want to add ¼ to ¼:

1. **Ensure that the bottom numbers (the denominators) are the same.**

   In this case they are (they're both 4) and so you can proceed to Step 2.

2. **Add the top numbers (the numerators) and put this answer over the denominator.**

   $1 + 1 = 2$, giving you the fraction ²⁄₄.

3. **Simplify the fraction (see the preceding section), if required.**

   2 goes into 2 once and into 4 twice, giving ½.

If the fraction has different denominators, such as ⅓ + ⅙, you need to make the denominators the same before you can continue from Step 1. To do so, in this case, you multiply the top and bottom of the first fraction by 2, because 3 goes into 6 two times.

$$1 \times 2 = 2$$
$$3 \times 2 = 6$$

This calculation gives you ²⁄₆. Now you're able to go Step 2: ²⁄₆ + ⅙ = ³⁄₆.

Simplifying the fraction (3 goes into 3 once and into 6 twice) gives you (drum roll, please) ½!

Taking away fractions

To subtract fractions, you use the same three basic steps as for adding them. Here, you want to work out ¾ – ¼:

1. **Ensure that the bottom numbers (the denominators) are the same.**

   They are (4) and so proceed to Step 2.

2. Subtract the top number (the numerator) and put this answer over the denominator.

$3 - 1 = 2$, giving you the fraction $\frac{2}{4}$.

3. Simplify the fraction, if required.

2 goes into 2 once and into 4 twice, giving $\frac{1}{2}$.

If the fraction has different denominators, such as $\frac{1}{2} - \frac{1}{6}$, you multiply the top and bottom of the first fraction by 3 in this case (because 2 goes into 6 three times).

$1 \times 3 = 3$

$2 \times 3 = 6$

This multiplication gives you $\frac{3}{6}$. Now you can carry out Step 2: $\frac{3}{6} - \frac{1}{6} = \frac{2}{6}$. Simplifying the fraction (2 goes into 2 once and into 6 three times) gives you $\frac{1}{3}$.

Multiplying and dividing fractions

Knowing how to multiply and divide fractions in healthcare is important. For example, you regularly divide fractions when calculating prescribed tablets. Say that Amoxicillin 500 milligrams three times a day is prescribed and 250-milligram Amoxicillin capsules are available. You need to work out the correct number of capsules to give for each dose ($\frac{500}{250} = 2$ capsules).

Multiplying

To multiply fractions, you simply multiply the numbers above the line together and then the numbers below the line. You can do so in three simple steps – why complicate things! Here you need to calculate $\frac{2}{5} \times \frac{4}{7}$:

1. Multiply the top numbers (the numerators).

$2 \times 4 = 8$.

2. Multiply the bottom numbers (the denominators).

$5 \times 7 = 35$.

3. Simplify if required.

You can't simplify the answer here ($\frac{8}{35}$).

Dividing

Here are the three steps to divide a fraction. In this case, you want to work out ⅔ ÷ ¼:

1. **Turn the second fraction (the one you need to divide by) upside down (called a *reciprocal*).**

   In this case, ¼ becomes ⁴/₁.

2. **Multiply the first fraction by the reciprocal.**

   ⅔ × ⁴/₁ = ⁸/₃.

3. **Simplify the fraction, if required.**

   Not possible for this example.

Converting fractions into decimals

Sometimes you may find that converting fractions into decimals is appropriate in the healthcare environment. For example, when looking in the British National Formulary you see that a drug costing £44.56 for a pack of 30 tablets can be obtained for ½ the price of this leading brand. What does ½ equate to? £44.56 divided by 2 = £22.28. (Check out Chapter 2 for an introduction to decimals.)

With a calculator

The quickest method of converting fractions into decimals is to use a calculator! Just get your top number and divide it by the bottom number to get the decimal number of your fraction. Bingo! For example:

- ⁵/₁₂ = 5 divided by 12 = 0.41666
- ²/₄ = 2 divided by 4 = 0.5
- ⁶/₉ = 6 divided by 9 = 0.6666
- ⅝ = 5 divided by 8 = 0.625

I think you get the picture. Table 3-1 shows the decimal numbers of some other fractions.

Table 3-1	Decimal Numbers of Common Fractions		
Fraction	*Simplified Fraction*	*In Words*	*Decimal*
$^{10}/_{100}$	$^{1}/_{10}$	One-tenth	0.1 (0.10)
$^{20}/_{100}$	$^{1}/_{5}$	One-fifth	0.2 (0.20)
$^{25}/_{100}$	¼	One-quarter	0.25
$^{33}/_{100}$	$^{1}/_{3}$	One-third	0.33
$^{50}/_{100}$	½	One-half	0.5 (0.50)
$^{66}/_{100}$	$^{2}/_{3}$	Two-thirds	0.6 (recurring)
$^{75}/_{100}$	¾	Three-quarters	0.75

Changing a fraction to a decimal manually

Here are the steps to change a fraction to a decimal manually, in this case ¾:

1. **Find a number by which you can multiply the fraction's denominator (the bottom number) to make it 10, 100 or 1,000 (or any number with a 1 followed by zeros).**

   In this case, you multiply the 4 by 25 to become 100.

2. **Multiply the numerator (the top) and the denominator by that number.**

   Here, 3 and 4 multiplied by 25 gives $^{75}/_{100}$.

3. **Write down the top number only, putting the decimal point in the correct spot (one space from the right-hand side for every zero in the bottom number).**

   In this case, you have 75.0, which with the decimal point moved 2 spaces to the left (because 100 has two zeros) gives your answer of 0.75.

Grappling with Decimals

Decimal numbers are all around you, in everyday life and in healthcare. Perhaps you've seen medications expressed as 3.5 milligrams. This number has a decimal point. All decimal numbers are based on the number 10, and so 3.5 means that you require less than the whole number: 3 units and 5 tenths.

This section leads you through working with decimals and fractions. Flip to Chapter 2 for much more on handling decimals.

As you move left from the decimal point, each digit is 10 times bigger.

Thinking about decimals and fractions

A *decimal fraction* has a value of less than 1, but more than 0. The following numbers are all decimal fractions:

- 0.3
- 0.1
- 0.999
- 0.656565

A *mixed number* is a combination of a whole number and a decimal fraction. These numbers are called *improper fractions* (they can be rude, burping all over the place!). Here are some examples, along with how you can think of them as fractions:

- **59.2:** 59 and $\frac{2}{10}$
- **20.86:** 20 and $\frac{86}{100}$
- **13.76:** 13 and $\frac{76}{100}$

You come across decimal fractions every day in healthcare. One common example is the body temperature recording of 36–37.5 degrees Celsius. Each degree is divided from the whole number into tenths, such as 36.1, 36.2, 36.3 and so on. Therefore, 37.5 is recoded as 37 degrees Celsius plus 5 tenths.

Rounding decimal numbers

Decimal numbers describe tenths, hundredths and thousandths of a number. For example, the number 7.98 is equal to one whole unit, plus a fraction or part of the number (0.98).

In healthcare, you sometimes have to round this part up or down to get a whole number. For instance, if you're setting up an intravenous infusion (check out Chapter 16), you can't count part of a drop – this figure has to be a whole. So, if you're counting a drip rate, the number can't be 4.8 drops: it has to be a 4 or a 5.

Using the rule of 5s

To achieve this goal, you use a principle called *the rule of 5s:*

✔ If the number after the decimal point is 4 or less, you round *down*.

✔ If the number after the decimal point is 5 or more, you round *up*.

For example, 44.4 rounds down to the whole number of 44 because the 0.4 part is below 5.

Here are more examples of numbers that have been rounded up or down to create a whole number:

✔ 44.72 = 45

✔ 39.3 = 39

✔ 0.99 = 1

✔ 1.55 = 2

✔ 2.3 = 2

✔ 3.21 = 3

As you can see, when you have more than one number after the decimal point, you still use the rule of fives. So, 33.27 becomes 33, because the number after the decimal point is 2, which is less than 5. However, the figure 49.66 becomes 50, because the number after the decimal point is 6, which is more than 5.

Rounding off to how many places?

When rounding off the decimal number, you need to decide whether you want to do so to one decimal place, two decimal places or three decimal places. You still use the rule of 5s, though:

✔ Rounding off to one decimal place:

- 2.65 = 2.7
- 1.04 = 1.0
- 0.47 = 0.5

✔ Rounding off to two decimal places:

- 0.625 = 0.63
- 1.571 = 1.57
- 2.428 = 2.43

 ✔ Rounding off to three decimal places:

- 0.1645 = 0.165

- 1.4145 = 1.415

- 3.0909 = 3.091

Converting decimals into fractions

To convert a decimal into a fraction (for example, when administering medication you usually express amounts as fractions not decimals), you first change the decimal into a whole number, by moving the decimal point to the right, and then you divide the denominator (the lower number) by a multiple of 10.

How many places you move the decimal point to the right is determined by the value of the multiple of 10 you require, which means how many zeros you have. For instance:

✔ **If you have a denominator of 10:** Move the decimal point 1 place to the right.

✔ **If you have a denominator of 100:** Move the decimal point 2 places to the right.

✔ **If you have a denominator of 1,000:** Move the decimal point 3 places to the right.

To determine what the denominator will be, you need to check how many decimal places you need to move the decimal to make a whole number – this gives you the number of zeros and then you add a 1 to the start of the zeros. For example, to convert 0.75 into a fraction, you move the point two points to the right to make 75 the fraction's numerator (top number). The denominator (the bottom number) is 100 because you must move the decimal point 2 times to make a whole number and then add the 1 to the start of the zeros: hence $^{75}/_{100}$.

You can simplify (see the earlier section 'Simplifying fractions') $^{75}/_{100}$ by dividing the numerator and the denominator by 25, because 25 goes into 75 three times and 25 goes into 100 four times: ¾.

Table 3-2 shows decimals converted to fractions, and then further simplified.

Table 3-2	Some Common Decimals as Fractions	
Decimal	*Fraction*	*Simplified Fraction*
0.1 (0.10)	$^{10}/_{100}$	$^1/_{10}$
0.2 (0.20)	$^{20}/_{100}$	$^1/_5$
0.25	$^{25}/_{100}$	¼
0.33	$^{33}/_{100}$	$^1/_3$
0.5 (0.50)	$^{50}/_{100}$	½
0.66	$^{66}/_{100}$	$^2/_3$
0.75	$^{75}/_{100}$	¾

If you have the fraction $^{25}/_{100}$ and want to know its decimal number, you can just use a calculator: simply input 25 divided by 100 and you get the decimal number of 0.25. If you also input the simplified fraction 1 divided by 4, you get 0.25, because the decimal number for the fraction $^{25}/_{100}$ and the simplified fraction ¼ is 0.25.

Turning decimals into percentages

A percentage is a number expressed as a fraction of 100. Fractions, decimals and percentages all represent parts of a whole. For example:

25% = 0.25 = ¼ = one quarter

In other words, a percentage is a way of expressing a number as a fraction of 100 (Chapter 4 covers percentages in more detail).

Percentages are used in healthcare in a variety of ways, such as intravenous fluid hydration where labels state information such as 'sodium chloride 0.9% w/v': w/v means weight in volume (see Chapter 5).

To work out the percentage of a decimal number, you can multiply it by 100 and then add the percentage sign. For example:

$0.1 \times 100 = 10\%$

$0.2 \times 100 = 20\%$

Alternatively, you can move the decimal point two places to the right, which is the same as multiplying the decimal number by 100. Simple!

Table 3-3 shows some more examples of decimals converted into percentage format.

Table 3-3	Some Common Decimals as Percentages
Decimal	*Percentage*
0.1 (0.10)	10%
0.2 (0.20)	20%
0.25	25%
0.33	33%
0.5 (0.50)	50%
0.66	66%
0.75	75%

Chapter 4

Ordering Parts with Percentages, Averages and Ratios

*Y*ou use percentages, averages and ratios regularly in your everyday life, whether you want to know how much of your monthly salary you spend on pizza or the average number of hours you spend watching TV, or you want to compare your couch-potato time with your hours spent working up a sweat in the gym. But however important pizza and TV are (very, of course), being competent handling these three mathematical areas is never more important than when working with patients in the healthcare setting.

This section guides you through doing so, for example when you're administrating medications or checking a patient's condition, so that you can complete the task confidently and keep your patients safe.

Peering into the World of Percentages

A *percentage* is a way of expressing a number as a portion of 100, or to put it another way, as a number of parts per hundred parts. In a sense percentages are the same as decimals and fractions (see Chapters 2 and 3, respectively), which also represent parts of a whole:

Percentage Value	Decimal Value	Fraction Value	In Words
50%	0.5	1/2	One half

Here are a few examples:

- ✔ **2.5%:** 2.5 parts per 100 parts
- ✔ **15%:** 15 parts per 100 parts
- ✔ **19%:** 19 parts per 100 parts
- ✔ **25%:** 25 parts per 100 parts
- ✔ **50%:** 50 parts per 100 parts
- ✔ **99%:** 99 parts per 100 parts

Therefore, at a quick glance you can see that '50%' means ½ of the whole and that '25%' means ¼ of the whole.

Using percentages in healthcare is a useful means of comparing different quantities: for example, when working out how much drug is in a solution at a quick glance.

When dealing with intravenous (IV) fluids, and being presented for example with a 1-litre bag of '0.9% sodium chloride w/v', you need to know exactly what this description means (w/v just means weight in volume, see Chapter 5 for more on this).

You work that out as follows:

1. **Change 1 litre into the millilitre (ml) format by multiplying by 1,000.**

   In this case, $1 \times 1,000 = 1,000$ ml (see Chapter 2 for all about converting units of measurement).

2. **Multiple the 1,000 ml by 0.9 divided by 100: $^{0.9}\%_{100} \times 1,000$ ml = 9 grams.**

   Therefore, the 1-litre bag contains 9 grams of sodium chloride.

If the bag had 500 ml of 0.9% sodium chloride, you'd know that it equates to 4.5 ml grams in the bags:

$$^{0.9}\%_{100} \times 500 \text{ ml} = 4.5 \text{ grams}$$

When using percentages in the healthcare setting, you need to know whether you're converting decimals to percentages, or percentages to decimals, calculating fractions into percentages, or even the percentage of a number. In other words, what do you want the percentage to be when it grows up?

Thinking about percentages and decimals

You need to know the mathematical principles of changing decimals into percentages or vice versa, so that if this skill is required in your specialism, you're fully capable of carrying out the task successfully and confidently.

A percentage can be less than 1 per cent. For example:

- 0.4% = 0.4 parts per 100 (or 4 parts per 1,000).
- 0.06% = 0.06 parts per 100 (or 6 parts per 10,000).

Converting decimals into a percentage format is just a case of multiplying by 100.

Here's how you change 0.5 into a percentage:

$$0.5 = (0.5 \times 100)\% = 50\%$$

Therefore, the decimal number 0.5 equates to 50 per cent.

To multiply by 100, you can move the decimal point two places to the right. To convert percentages into decimals, you simply divide by 100.

To change 30 per cent into a decimal:

$$30\% = 30 \div 100 = 0.3$$

Therefore, 30 per cent is the same as 0.3 in its decimal format.

To divide by 100, you can move the decimal point two places to the left.

Converting fractions into percentages

In healthcare, you can find that expressing numbers in percentages rather than in fractions is easier. For instance, for a patient who has had $\frac{4}{10}$ of his daily oral fluid intake today, you'd be better expressing this as 40 per cent when discussing the situation with other healthcare professionals.

To convert a fraction into a percentage, you simply multiply by 100. If you need to do the reverse – convert a percentage into a fraction – you simply divide by 100 (bet you saw that one coming!).

Take a look at changing these fractions into percentages:

- ✔ $^4/_{10}$: $(4 \times 100) / 10\% = 40\%$
- ✔ $^2/_5$: $(2 \times 100) / 5\% = 40\%$
- ✔ $^1/_2$: $(1 \times 100) / 2\% = 50\%$
- ✔ $^3/_6$: $(3 \times 100) / 6\% = 50\%$
- ✔ $^2/_8$: $(2 \times 100) / 8\% = 25\%$
- ✔ $^1/_6$: $(1 \times 100) / 6\% = 16.666 = 17$ to the nearest whole number

Calculating the percentage of a number

To work out the percentage of a number, you can use this formula:

Number $/ 100 \times$ percentage required

For example, to work out 40 per cent of 3,088:

$$^{3,088}/_{100} \times 40\% = 1,235.2 = 1,235 \text{ (to the nearest whole number)}$$

Here are six more examples of finding the percentage of a number, to get you really into the swing of things!

- ✔ **54% of 510:** $^{510}/_{100} \times 54\% = 275.4$ (275 to the nearest whole number)
- ✔ **89% of 25:** $^{25}/_{100} \times 89\% = 22.25 = $ (22 to the nearest whole number)
- ✔ **60% of 80:** $^{80}/_{100} \times 60\% = 48$
- ✔ **17% of 9,120:** $^{9,120}/_{100} \times 17\% = 1,550.4 = $ (1,550 to the nearest whole number)
- ✔ **2% of 4,524:** $^{4,524}/_{100} \times 2\% = 90.48 = $ (90 to the nearest whole number)
- ✔ **40% of 27,000,000:** $^{27,000,000}/_{100} \times 40\% = 10,800,000$

Getting percentages from percentages

Sometimes you may need to work out one percentage amount from another. For example, imagine that you're asked to find the percentage of the following situation:

In a calculations test, 290 student nurses out of 400 passed this test the first time.

Here's the formula to get the answer:

Smaller number / Larger number × 100

So, your calculation goes as follows:

$^{290}/_{400} \times 100 = 72.5 = 73\%$ (to the nearest whole number)

Of course, you can reverse this answer and state that 27 per cent failed the test the first time! But why focus on the negative!

As with all calculations, look at the whole picture and see whether the answer makes sense and looks right: 290 out of 400 students passed the calculations test and so 73 per cent looks about right.

A medication costing £15.75 for 100 millilitres has had a price increase of 10 per cent. You work out the new cost of the medication as follows:

$^{15.75}/_{100} \times 10 = 1.57.$

You then add this amount (£1.57) to the original cost (£15.75) to get £17.32. The healthcare setting may now consider this price rise too much and revert to using a cheaper brand.

Administering drug amounts involving percentages

Many intravenous (IV) fluids contain percentages, for example:

- **5% dextrose:** Meaning 5 grams of dextrose per 100 millilitres of solution.

- **0.9% sodium chloride:** Meaning 0.9 per cent sodium chloride per 100 millilitres of solution, or:
  - 4.5 grams of sodium chloride per 500 millilitres of solution
  - 9 grams of sodium chloride per 1,000 millilitres (1 litre) of solution

Adjusting percentages for individual patients

Sometimes you're required to work out a percentage around a patient's nutritional requirements or medication changes.

The doctor wants a patient to decrease his 160 millilitres of medication by 15 per cent. By how many millilitres does this amount need to be decreased, and how much of the medication does the patient still have to take? The question is asking you to work out a percentage from a number (see the earlier 'Calculating the percentage of a number' section), and so you can use this formula to come to the amount by which to decrease the medication:

$$^{160}\!/_{100} \times 15\% = {}^{8}\!/_{5} \times 15 = 24 \text{ ml}$$

So from the 160 millilitres in the patient's bottle of medication, you can waste 24 millilitres, leaving the patient with 136 millilitres of medication still left to take (160 − 24 = 136 ml).

Using percentages with the injectables

Percentages are often used in healthcare in reports and research articles. A midwife may relate to a new mother that at the end of week one, her baby has lost 12 per cent of his original birth weight and suggest 'top up' formula feeds between breast feeds. By the end of the second week the loss is just 6 per cent and by the end of week 3, baby has gained weight and now is back to the birth weight.

Percentages can also present themselves in calculations involving the local anaesthetic lidocaine hydrochloride injections and other injectable drugs.

Lidocaine hydrochloride is absorbed effectively from the mucous membranes and is useful as a surface anaesthetic in concentrations up to and not exceeding 10 per cent.

Imagine that a patient has to have a rogue mole removed from his abdomen and sent to pathology to check to see whether it's cancerous. Now I don't know about you, but if I'm having a bit of my body cut away, however small, I want all the numbing effects I can get! What I don't want is to be overdosed and experience any toxic effects.

Lidocaine is produced in concentrations of 0.5, 1 and 2 per cent. The dose is based on the patient's weight with a maximum recommended dose of 200 milligrams.

You're asked to administer '10 ml of a 1% solution': how many milligrams does your patient require? 1 per cent solution means 1 gram of the drug in every 100 millilitres, and so after changing your 1 gram into 1,000 millilitres, you can check the dose as follows:

$$^{1,000 \text{ mg}}\!/_{100 \text{ ml}} = {}^{10 \text{ mg}}\!/_{1 \text{ ml}}$$

Therefore, each 1 millilitre equates to 10 milligrams of the drug. You need to give 10 millilitres of the drug, which equals 100 milligrams and doesn't exceed the maximum dose of 200 milligrams.

1 per cent of lidocaine equates to 10 mg/ml, and so you know that 2 per cent of lidocaine equals 20 mg/ml and 5 per cent equals 50 mg/ml.

Children require much smaller doses of lidocaine, because for medication purposes they're really little people:

Lidocaine	*Microgram per millilitre*
0.1%	1,000 micrograms
0.2%	2,000 micrograms
0.5%	5,000 micrograms

Appreciating the Usefulness of Averages

Within healthcare, averages are statistics collected as a means of studying data, perhaps when reading pieces of research or when collecting data from your patients in relation to their physiological measurements by taking their observations. From this data, you're comparing your findings with the normal range, from which you can draw conclusions, such as:

> *Oh my goodness, my patient is really unwell, his temperature is well above the normal range. Better get some paracetamol prescribed!*

I introduce you to the four types of averages you encounter in healthcare and use a couple of practical examples to walk you through them. Prepare to meet hospital patients Lester and Teddy.

Defining and working with different averages

When you talk about averages, you can be talking about four different types:

- **Mean:** The number you get when all the values are added together and divided by the number of units.

- **Median:** Where you place all the numbers in order of size and use the number that's placed in the centre.

✔ **Mode:** The value that occurs most often.

✔ **Range:** Where you look at the difference between the highest and lowest values in a set of numbers.

To lead you through these four types, I use the pulse rate recordings of adult patient Lester as shown in Table 4-1 (to revise your understanding of the 24-hour clock, check out Chapter 6).

Table 4-1	Patient's Pulse Rate over a 16-hour Period
Time Pulse Taken	*Pulse Rate (Beats Per Minute)*
06:00	68
08:00	84
10:00	82
12 noon	90
14:00	86
16:00	90
18:00	72
20:00	70
22:00	64

Mean averages

This average type is the most common measure of average data that you tend to use. To find the mean average, you add all the numbers together and divide the total by the amount of numbers.

Mean = sum of numbers ÷ amount of numbers:

$$64 + 68 + 70 + 72 + 82 + 84 + 86 + 90 + 90 = 706$$

$$706 \div 9 = 78.4$$

Therefore, Lester's mean average pulse rate is 78 (to the nearest whole number).

Median averages

The median average is the number in the middle, when you place all the numbers in numerical order, as follows:

64	68	70	72	82	84	86	90	90

You can see that 82 is in the middle and therefore 82 is Lester's median average pulse rate.

If you have two middle numbers in your list, the median is the mean of those two numbers.

Mode averages

This average type is the number that occurs most frequently in the data. If you look at Table 4-1, you can see that Lester's mode average pulse rate is 90 (which appears twice).

Range averages

The range average is the difference between the highest number and the lowest number in a set of numbers. To find it, you subtract the lowest number from the highest:

64	68	70	72	82	84	86	90	90

$90 - 64 = 26$

Therefore, the range for Lester's pulse rate is 26.

Putting averages to work in healthcare

You use averages all the time in healthcare, from looking at 'average' nurses' pay articles in daily newspapers (and sighing heavily), to viewing research papers and looking at statistics.

More often, however, you use them to get information regarding your patient's medical condition, such as measuring his intra-cranial pressure recordings, and administering the correct medical intervention required from the data received.

You need to find the mean average for patient Teddy, who's in critical care after being involved in a traffic accident. He received a traumatic head injury and is presently in a comatose state. His intra-cranial pressure (ICP) recordings (measured in milligrams of mercury – known as mmHg, a unit of pressure measurement) for a 2-hour period are as follows:

- ✔ 14:00: 18.0 mmHg
- ✔ 14:30: 18.0 mmHg
- ✔ 15:00: 18.5 mmHg
- ✔ 15:30: 19.0 mmHg
- ✔ 16:00: 17.0 mmHg

From a purely mathematical prospective, you don't need to know what the heck a 'intra-cranial pressure recording' is, because you just need to know the mean average: the sum of the values divided by the number of units. Of course, if you work in critical care, you most certainly need to know all about this!

1. **Add up the readings as follows:**

   $18.0 + 18.0 + 18.5 + 19 + 17.0 = 90.5$

2. **Divide by the number of readings taken:**

   $90.5 \div 5 = 18.1$ mmHg (Teddy's mean average ICP recording)

Reading about Ratios

Many nurses have told me, 'I hate ratios'! 'Why,' I reply over the sound of pounding music. 'What have radios ever done to you?' No, ratios,' they shout. Perhaps I shouldn't play the Radio 2 breakfast show so loud, but my question stands: what have ratios ever done to you?

Ratios are simply a means of comparing two quantities. These quantities need to be in the same format of units. The following sections take a closer look at ratios and what you need to know.

Defining ratios

A *ratio* is a way of comparing amounts of something. For example, imagine that a ward has 20 patients and two nurses agree to split them '50:50' (not literally, that would be painful for them and rather messy for the nurses!). As a result, one nurse takes charge and delivers care to 10 patients and the other nurse takes charge and delivers care to the other 10 patients. Nice teamwork!

If one of the nurses suggests that he'll take charge of 5 of the patients and asks you to take charge of the other 15 patients, the split would be 5:15. Or, put more simply, 1:3, meaning that you're caring for three times the amount of patients than your lazy colleague!

As you can see, a ratio tells you the size of parts of anything that can be shared out.

Using ratios in healthcare

Ratios are all around healthcare staff, and not just when administering medication.

I discuss two different formats of ratios:

- ✔ **Part to part ratios:** Written with a colon, for example '1:4', and meaning 1 part to 4 parts (thus a total of 5 parts). This ratio example may be used to express how much diluent needs to be added to a concentrated oral drug: for example, contrast medium to aid visibility where a patient requires an X-ray.

- ✔ **Part to whole ratios:** Written as, for example '1 in 4', to mean 1 part in a total of 4 parts. This ratio example may be used in skin care for patients with weeping eczema. A doctor may prescribe 400 milligrams of potassium permanganate for bathing in a concentration of 1 in 10,000 solution. A 1 in 10,000 solution is 0.1 milligram per 1 millilitre: $\frac{400 \text{ mg}}{0.1 \text{ mg}} \times 1 \text{ ml} = 4{,}000 \text{ ml} = 4$ litres. Therefore the 400-milligram tablet would need to be diluted in 4 litres of water – a very diluent concentration.

Therefore, *1:4* equates to *1 in 5* and *1:3* equates to *1 in 4*. Confused? You won't be after you read this section!

Gasping to see part to part ratios in practice

Imagine that you're making up jugs of squash for patients to drink during a heatwave. The 500-millilitre bottle of concentrated fruit juice states 'Dilute 7 parts of water to 1 part of juice'. The ward sister asks you how much juice can be made from the bottle. The way that the task is presented to you means that you look for a part to part ratio (with a colon).

You know that each 1 part is worth 500 millilitres (the juice amount), and so this amount equates to 1:7, meaning that you have eight parts in total $(1 + 7 = 8)$:

$$500 \times 1 = 500$$

$$500 \times 7 = 3{,}500$$

$$3{,}500 + 500 = 4{,}000 \text{ ml in total}$$

Alternatively, 500 ml $\times$ 8 = 4,000 ml (or 4 litres)

Therefore, you add 3,500 ml of water to make the whole liquid amount of 4,000 ml of juice to satisfy your thirsty patients.

Imagine that an audit is being conducted in a clinical area into how many female patients are completing the 'friends and family test' survey as opposed to male patients. Female patients have completed 15 completed forms and the male patients 12 today. You're asked to send the results to the clinical audit office as a ratio, in the simplest form.

You can see that the part for part ratio of females to males is 15:12.

Both sides of the ratio are divisible by 3, giving you 5:4, neither of which has a common factor (apart from the number 1). Therefore, the simplest form of this ratio is 5:4. Five females completed this survey for every 4 males.

Here are some examples of solution ratios expressed in the part for part ratio format:

- Ratio of 1:4 of a stock solution of 100 ml = 20 ml ($1 + 4 = 5$; $100 \div 5$)
- Ratio of 1:9 of a stock solution of 5 litres = 500 ml ($1 + 9 = 10$; $5{,}000 \div 10$)
- Ratio of 1:10 of a stock solution of 550 ml = 50 ml ($1 + 10 = 11$; $550 \div 11$)
- Ratio of 1:3 of a stock solution of 600 ml = 150 ml ($1 + 3 = 4$; $600 \div 4$)

Seeing part to whole ratios in action

You also come across ratios when dealing with solutions and concentrates. In this case you can express the ratio in the part to whole format: as '1 in 4', meaning 1 part stock solution added in 3 parts of diluted solution, making a total of 4 parts.

Adrenalin ratios

Adrenalin (epinephrine) is a drug given in emergency situations, such as anaphalaxis or circulatory failure.

- Adrenalin for anaphylaxis is expressed as 1:1,000, meaning 1 milligram for every 1 millilitre (1 mg/ml). Therefore, if you need to administer 0.5 milligrams of the drug, you give 0.5 millilitres.

- Adrenalin for cardiac arrest is expressed as 1:10,000, meaning 1 milligram in 10 millilitres (or 0.1 mg for every 1 ml). As you administer the whole 10 millilitres of the drug in this situation, you're giving ten times the volume than for the anaphylaxis situation.

As you can see, you really need to remember that 1 in 4 *isn't* the same as 1:4. 1 in 4 is a total of 4 parts and 1:4 is a total of 5 parts.

The ratio of 1 in 10 means 1 part stock solution to every 9 parts of dilutent: 10 parts in total. 10 − 1 = 9 parts of dilutent, therefore 1 in 10 equates to 1:9.

Check out these examples of ratios expressed in this format:

- Ratio of 1 in 4 of a stock solution of 100 ml = 25 ml (100 ÷ 4)
- Ratio of 1 in 9 of a stock solution of 5 litres = 555.55, rounded up to 556 ml (5,000 ÷ 9)
- Ratio of 1 in 10 of a stock solution of 550 ml = 55 ml (550 ÷ 10)
- Ratio of 1 in 3 of a stock solution of 600 ml = 200 ml (600 ÷ 3)

Chapter 5

Making Sense of Moles and Solution Concentrates

. . . .

In This Chapter

▶ Understanding moles and millimoles

▶ Working with solution concentrates

. . . .

I discuss moles and solution concentrates in this chapter, because you often come across them in healthcare and you have to know what they mean when you see them.

I need to get one thing clear – the moles aren't furry burrowing creatures or a cluster of *melanocytes* (as in freckles)! These *moles* are a unit of mass measurement within the *Systeme Internationale* (SI, which I introduce in Chapter 2). They're used in chemistry to count the mass weight of atoms and molecules, such as electrolytes (see Chapter 15).

Unlike moles, solution concentrates are exactly as advertised. A *concentrated solution* is one with a larger amount of solute dissolved in a solution (known as the *solvent*). This is in contrast to dilute solutions, which have a smaller amount of the solute dissolved in the solution (which is usually, but not always, water).

Meeting Moles and Millimoles

As a nurse, you're required to administer drugs and medicines to patients in a variety of different measurement units. Clearly, you need to know what these units are and what they indicate, and you have to be able to convert between different measuring systems – which is why you're sure to find the info in this section invaluable.

Defining moles

Moles are quite large units, and so millimoles are more commonly used in healthcare. You encounter millimoles when looking at biochemistry blood test results, such as sodium levels. Sodium and the other electrolytes are measured in millimoles:

- ✔ 1 mole is the equivalent of 1,000 millimoles.

- ✔ 1 millimole is the equivalent of 1,000 *micromoles* (mcmol). You can also express micro with the symbol μ, and so 1 micromole = 1 μmol.

You don't normally use the abbreviations for micromoles, however, due to the risk of confusion with millimoles and hence errors occurring.

Chemists may prefer to use the SI units of moles and millimoles to measure quantities of certain substances, because doing so can be more accurate than using the larger SI unit of grams.

The *mole* (mol) is a measurement of the relative atomic mass of a substance in grams. To break that down, everything is made up of atoms. Elements are atoms of the same kind. Water is made up of the elements hydrogen (H) and oxygen, with the chemical symbol of water being: H_2O. This means that it's made up of two atoms of hydrogen and one of oxygen. Every element has its own relative atomic mass – weight. Welcome to the world of mole!

Many of the patients' biochemistry results are presented as millimoles per litre of blood, such as electrolyte levels in blood samples. Anything out of the normal range tends to require medical intervention. Table 5-1 shows some of these laboratory results, with their normal ranges.

Table 5-1	Biochemistry Normal Parameters		
Test Name	*Units*	*Range (Low)*	*Range (High)*
Sodium	mmol/l	133	146
Potassium	mmol/l	3.5	5.3
Urea	mmol/l	2.5	7.8
Chloride	mmol/l	95	108
Bicarbonate	mmol/l	22	29
Phosphate	mmol/l	0.8	1.5
Magnesium	mmol/l	0.7	1.0

Test Name	Units	Range (Low)	Range (High)
Osmolality	mmol/kg	275	295
Alkaline Phosphatase (ALP)	units/litre	30	130
Creatine Kinase (CK)	units/litre		
Male		40	320
Female		25	200
Bilirubin (total)	μmol/l		≤21
Adjusted Calcium	mmol/l	2.2	2.6
Urate	μmol/l		
Male		200	430
Female		140	360
Carbamazepine	mg/l	4	12
Phenobarbitone	mg/l	10	40
Phenytoin	mg/l	5	20
Lithium	mmol/l	0.4	1.0
24-hour urine urate	mmol/24h	1.5	4.5
24-hour urine phosphate	mmol/24h	15	50
24-hour urine magnesium	mmol/24h	2.4	6.5
Albumen	g/l	36	46
Cholesterol (total) fasting	mmol/l		≤5.2
Globin	g/l	26	40
Iron	μmol/l		
Male		14	30
Female		9.0	26
PCO_2 (arterial)	kPa*	4.5	6.0
PO_2 (arterial)	kPa*	11.2	14.5
Protein (total)	g/l	60	80
Zinc	μmol/l	11	21
Glucose (fasting)	mmol/l	3.5	5.5

*kPa is a unit of pressure measurement, known as kilopascal: 1 kPa = 1,000 Pascals (Pa). It has largely replaced the pounds per square inch (psi) worldwide, which is used in the imperial measurement system.

Converting moles into millimoles

To convert the higher amount of substance – the mole – into the equivalent millimole, you need to know the basic decimal principle as follows (to check your understanding of 1 mole and 1 millimole equivalents, flip to the preceding section):

   ✔ **To convert from a larger unit to a smaller unit:** Multiply by multiples of 1,000.

   ✔ **To convert from a smaller unit to a larger unit:** Divide by multiples of 1,000.

Imagine that you need to convert 1 mole into 1 millimole. In other words you're changing a higher unit (the mole) into a smaller unit (the millimole). The equation is simply $1 \times 1,000 = 1,000$ millimoles.

Changing millimoles into milligrams per litre

Patients with diabetes require regular blood glucose monitoring. Performing this test on patients is one of the most common bedside activities.

The aim is always to maintain blood glucose levels usually between the ranges of 4 and 7 millimoles, as far as possible.

The chemical formula for glucose is: $C_6H_{12}O_6$, which means that the relative atomic mass weights of each of the elements are: carbon = 6, hydrogen = 12 and oxygen = 6.

The molecular weight (or relative molecular mass) of glucose is 180 grams: that is, 1 mole of glucose weighs 180 grams.

Therefore, you can change millimoles in milligrams per litre as follows:

   ✔ 4 mmol/l is equivalent to $4 \times 180 = 720$ mg/l

   ✔ 5 mmol/l is equivalent to $5 \times 180 = 900$ mg/l

   ✔ 6 mmol/l is equivalent to $6 \times 180 = 1,080$ mg/l

   ✔ 7 mmol/l is equivalent to $7 \times 180 = 1,260$ mg/l

Concentrating on Solution Concentrates

Many medicines come in the form of a *solution,* which contains a *solute* (the original substance) dissolved in a *solvent* (often liquid). A *concentration* refers to the amount of solute that's dissolved in the solvent.

The solution can be dilute or concentrated:

- ✔ **Dilute solution:** Contains particularly small amounts of dissolved minerals. An everyday example is tap water.
- ✔ **Concentrated solution:** Contains large amounts of the solute in a smaller volume of solvent. An example is the opioid Oramorph concentrated oral solution 20mg/ml. Each Oramorph concentrated solution contains 20 mg of morphine sulphate.

You can express drug strengths in a number of ways in order to work out how much of the actual pharmaceutical product is present in a medicine. In this section I describe different ways of indicating concentrations. I promise no dilution of facts; just all concentrated informative goody-goodness!

Perusing percentage concentrates

One way of describing the solution concentrate is to use the percentage as a unit. Here are three common ways of doing so:

- ✔ **% weight in volume:** Number of grams in 100 millilitres (ml)
- ✔ **% weight in weight:** Number of grams in 100 grams
- ✔ **% volume in volume:** Number of ml in 100 ml

Read on to discover more about each type.

Weight in volume: w/v

Sometimes, percentage concentrates are defined as the amount of drug in 100 parts of the product – in healthcare, most commonly expressed as *weight in volume* (w/v). This expression is used when a solid is dissolved in a liquid and it means the number of grams dissolved in 100 millilitres.

Check out these examples:

- ✔ Sodium chloride 0.9% w/v in 100 ml = 0.9/100 × 1 = 0.9%, in a 100-ml bag of fluid
- ✔ Sodium chloride 0.9% w/v in 1 l = 0.9/100 × 1,000 = 9 g, in a l-bag of fluid

- ✔ Glucose 5% in w/v 100 ml = 5/100 × 100 = 5 g, in a 100-ml bag of fluid

- ✔ Glucose 5% in w/v 1 l = 5/100 × 1,000 = 50 g, in a litre bag of fluid

- ✔ Sodium bicarbonate 8.4% w/v in 100 ml = 8.4/100 × 100 = 8.4 g, in a 100-ml bag of fluid

- ✔ Sodium bicarbonate 8.4% w/v in 200 ml = 8.4/100 × 200 = 16.8 g, in a 200-ml bag of fluid

Weight in weight: w/w

You can also come across percentage concentration as the *weight in weight* (w/w). This term is most commonly used for creams and ointments when a solid is mixed with another solid. Simply put, w/w means the number of grams in 100 grams.

A soap substitute antimicrobial and emollient treatment for eczema and dermatitis states on the patient information leaflet that the active ingredients of the lotion are as follows (I explain each item after the bold ingredient):

- ✔ **Benzalkonium chloride (0.1% w/w):** 0.1 g of benzalkonium chloride in 100 g

- ✔ **Chlorhexidine dihydrochloride (0.1% w/w):** 0.1 g of chlorhexidine dihydrochloride in 100 g

- ✔ **Liquid paraffin (2.5% w/w):** 2.5 g of liquid paraffin in 100 g

- ✔ **Isopropyl myristate (2.5% w/w):** 2.5 g of isopropyl myristate in 100 g

Volume in volume (v/v)

The third type of percentage concentration is *volume in volume* (v/v) – the number of millilitres in 100 millilitres – which is used when one liquid is mixed or diluted with another liquid.

When a medication is presented as '10% v/v', it indicates that 10 millilitres of the active ingredient is present in 100 millilitres of fluid.

When you next pick up a bottle of wine (for a friend, of course) look at the label. You'll notice that it states the concentration expressed as v/v%. Wine has about 12 millilitres of alcohol (ethanol) per 100 millilitres of solution. You can use the formula:

Solute volume (ml)/solution volume (ml) × 100 to find the solute concentration:

12 ml alcohol/100 ml solution × 100 = 12 v/v% alcohol.

Just to note, alcohol is often presented as 'proof'. The proof value is twice the v/v% value. Therefore, the wine above has a proof value of 24%.

Considering concentration strengths

Sometimes you see concentrations prescribed as '1 in . . .', which are also known as *ratio strengths*.

An example of this concentration expression is adrenalin 1 in 1,000 – used in the treatment of anaphylaxis (see Chapter 13). It means that the active ingredient (adrenalin) equates to 1 gram in 1,000 millilitres. Therefore, to administer 1 milligram you give 1 millilitre by subcutaneous or intramuscular injection.

The higher the number, the weaker the solution. For example, adrenalin is also available as 1 in 10,000, indicating 1 gram in 10,000 millilitres, which is weaker than 1 in 1,000.

Solving the solution of milligrams/ millilitre concentrations

The most common method of expressing the amount of drug in a solution is milligrams in millilitres (mg/ml).

In essence, mg/ml is saying how much of a drug in milligrams is present per millilitre of liquid (sometimes referred to as the *transport medium*):

✔ **For oral drugs:** Usually expressed as the number of mg in a standard 5-ml spoonful: for example, amoxicillin 250 mg in 5 ml. So, for every 5-ml spoonful, the patient is taking 250 mg of the drug; two spoonfuls and she's taking 500 mg of the drug.

✔ **For injections:** Usually expressed as the number of mg per volume of the ampoule (1 ml, 2 ml, 5 ml, 10 ml or 20 ml). For example:

• Loop diuretic furosemide (prescribed for pulmonary oedema, chronic heart failure and resistant hypertension) can be presented as 10 mg/ml, or 20 mg/2 ml, 50 mg/5 ml, 250 mg/25 ml.

• Gentamicin (prescribed for septicaemia and neonatal sepsis, meningitis, acute pyelonephritis, endocarditis and pneumonia) can be presented as 80 mg in 2 ml or 40 mg/2 ml.

Uniting the explanation of units

The strength of certain substances, such as insulin, is expressed in units of activity per given volume – for instance, 100 units per 1 ml – and is prescribed in units, such as '10 units actrapid insulin'.

Patients having problems with blood clotting or a thrombosis (blood clots) are most likely be prescribed heparin, which like insulin is prescribed in units of variable strengths, for example:

✔ **1,000 units/ml:**

- In ampoules of 1 ml, 5 ml, 10 ml, 20 ml

- In vials of 5 ml

✔ **5,000 units/1 l:**

- In ampoules of 1 ml, 5 ml

- In vials of 5 ml

✔ **25,000 units/ml:**

- In ampoules of 1 ml

- In vials of 5 ml

Many healthcare professionals have made drug errors by drawing up the wrong strength and administering the wrong dose of heparin.

To work out the prescribed amount of heparin to give to a patient by subcutaneous injection, use the following formula:

$$\text{What you want}\Big/\text{What you've got} \times \text{Volume}$$

If the patient is prescribed 15,000 units of heparin and you have vials containing 25,000 units/1 ml, you work this dose out as follows:

$$\frac{15,000}{25,000} \times 1 \text{ ml} = 0.6 \text{ ml}$$

The 0.6 ml dose is less than 1 ml and so you draw it up in a 1-ml syringe to ensure that you have the accurate dose.

Administering LMWH doses correctly

Heparin is an anticoagulant drug and comes in two forms: unfractionated heparin and low-molecular-weight heparin (LMWH). The latter differs from unfractionated heparin in its size and weight of molecules. (Unfractionated heparin molecules haven't been fractionated into LMWH.) Low-molecular-weight heparin can be given as a prophylaxis agent against thrombosis and as a subcutaneous injection. It's administered via a continuous syringe driver pump, after administering a loading dose of the heparin, by subcutaneous injection.

This drug can come in the following format:

20,000 units/20 ml in vials of 20 ml

Owing to the danger of overprescribing this medication, which is often used to reduce blood clot formation, you need to test the patient's blood on a daily basis and titrate the heparin according to these readings.

Chapter 6

Administering Drugs Accurately and Safely

*N*urses and healthcare staff handle and deal with drugs every working day. Patient safety has to be the number-one priority for all concerned.

Here I describe how to administer drugs safely and in line with the official guidelines, detailing the different methods and options you encounter. I also present a guide to interpreting what doctors write on patient prescription charts to help you avoid misunderstandings, including what they shouldn't do, but often do do!

Keeping Drug Safety in Mind

Registered General Nurses and Midwives are accountable for their actions and omissions when administering any medicines. They also have to comply with the Nursing and Midwifery Council Code of Conduct – known as 'The Code' (2015) and Medicines Management (2007) principles.

However, mistakes do happen: after all, 'to err is human'. To paraphrase Winston Churchill, everyone makes mistakes, but only wise people learn from them.

All healthcare staff need to learn from their mistakes and act on them so that the same mistakes don't continue to happen.

Research identifies two key areas of drug error:

- ✔ **Human factors:** One of the buzz phrases within healthcare at present – you may already have had a lecture about it! Human factors recognise that human error is normal, because humans aren't robots, and that therefore systems should be designed to allow for this reality and minimise risk.

  Human factors include environmental, organisational and job factors, and human and individual characteristics, which influence behaviour at work in ways that can affect health and safety.

- ✔ **Never events:** Another key phrase you may hear. Never events are preventable mistakes as categorised by the Department of Health: they should never have happened. In other words, where the potential exists for errors, tying up any loops to prevent mistakes before they occur.

More specifically, the National Patient Safety Agency (which receives data from healthcare organisations) issued a Safety Alert (for immediate action by all NHS organisations and one that concerns the independent sector) concerning the 'Safer Administration of Insulin':

> *[Concerning] the use of abbreviations such as U or IU (international units) for Units. When abbreviations are added to the intended dose, the dose may misread e.g. 10U is read as 100.*

> *The term units is to be used in all contexts. Abbreviations such as U or IU are never used.*

> *A training programme [is to be] put in place for all healthcare staff (including medical staff) expected to prescribe, prepare and administer insulin.*

For more on this problem, flip to the later section 'Knowing the abbreviations found on the prescription chart'.

Avoiding drug administration errors

Errors when administering medication can be due to a whole host of factors, including:

 ✔ Increasing demands on the nurse (or the person administering the medication)

 ✔ Low staffing levels

 ✔ Tiredness and stress

 ✔ Calculation errors

 ✔ Doctors handwriting being illegible on the prescription chart

 ✔ Doctors using Latin abbreviations on the prescription chart

 ✔ Complacency

 ✔ Distractions

 ✔ Confusing names of drugs that look and sound alike

 ✔ Lack of staff training

All healthcare workers need to apply professionalism and vigilance whenever administering medication. Before doing so, make sure that you know the adverse effects of the medicine and contraindications of the drug, as well as correct dosages for administration. To find this information, consult the latest British National Formulary (www.bnf.org), which is also available for children's drug information.

Many foods interact on drug metabolism and you need to know this information as well. Here are just four such interactions:

 ✔ **Garlic:** Interacts with anticoagulants.

 ✔ **Ginseng:** Interacts with warfarin, heparin, aspirin.

 ✔ **Grapefruit juice:** Interacts with nifedipine, nimodipine, carbamazepine, midazolam.

 ✔ **Soya:** Interacts with haloperidol, phenytoin, warfarin.

Check out the nearby sidebar 'Identifying the specific drugs that interact with some foods' for more on the drugs.

In addition, foods containing tyramine (found in mature cheese, pickled herring meat and yeast-extract spreads) can interact with *monoamine oxidase inhibitors* (MAOIs), drugs that are used in the treatment of depression, phobias, hypochondria and hysteria.

Identifying the specific drugs that interact with some foods

These drugs interact with garlic, ginseng and grapefruit juice:

✔ **Carbamazepine:** Prescribed for the prevention generalised tonic-clonic seizures, trigeminal neuralgia, bipolar disorder, acute alcohol withdrawal and diabetic neuropathy.

✔ **Haloperidol:** Prescribed for the treatment of schizophrenia, the control of tics and Tourette's syndrome.

✔ **Midazolam:** Prescribed for conscious sedation for procedures, sedation and status epilepticus.

✔ **Nifedipine:** Prescribed for hypertension, prophylaxis for angina and Raynaud's phenomenon.

✔ **Nimodipine:** Prescribed for the prevention and treatment of ischaemic neurological deficits.

✔ **Phenytoin:** Prescribed for status epilepticus and all forms of epilepsy except absence seizures and trigeminal neuralgia.

Dangers also exist if patients don't receive their medication in a timely fashion or they miss a dose. Figure 6-1's graph shows how the therapeutic blood serum levels can be disrupted due to a missed dose, and the importance of patient education. In this case, the clear advice is *not* to take two tablets to make up for a forgotten dose; doing so can cause toxicity and harm and the patient may overdose on the medication. Instead, patients should seek medical advice.

Figure 6-1: Graph showing the unwanted effect of trying to make up a missed medicine dose.

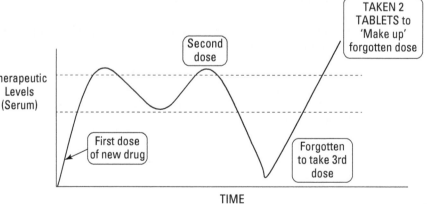

© John Wiley & Sons, Inc.

Remembering the rights of drug administration

You should always seek to administer medications to patients in a safe and professional manner. But mistakes can, and do, happen.

In order to minimise these errors, check out the following *Five Rights of Medication Administration* each time before administering a medication. I always go through this list as a mantra each time I'm administering drugs:

- ✔ Right drug
- ✔ Right patient
- ✔ Right dose
- ✔ Right route
- ✔ Right time

To help you remember, use this mnemonic: 'Don't let Patients Drink Raw Tuna'.

These five rights have also been expanded to the *Ten Rights of Medication Administration* in many healthcare areas:

- ✔ Right drug
- ✔ Right patient
- ✔ Right dose
- ✔ Right route
- ✔ Right time
- ✔ Right documentation
- ✔ Right client education
- ✔ Right to refuse
- ✔ Right assessment
- ✔ Right evaluation

Perhaps you can come up with your own mnemonic to help remember this longer list!

Spotting the difference between a drug and a medicine

Technically speaking, a difference exists between drugs and medicines, although people tend to refer to medicines as 'drugs' in the healthcare environment. I don't worry about the difference in this book, but so that you know, strictly speaking the distinction is as follows:

- ✔ **Drugs:** Substances that, when taken into the body, affect the structure or function of the living organism.

- ✔ **Medicines:** Drugs used in the treatment, diagnosis or prevention of a disease. All medicines have a Product Licence (PL) number indicating that they've been through clinical trials and are now licensed to be sold as a medicine. Without a PL number, the drug isn't a medicine.

Here are the four legal categories of medicine:

- ✔ **GSL (General Sales List) medicines:** People can buy these medicines in supermarkets and other small retail outlets in small amounts.

- ✔ **Pharmacy medicines:** A wider selection of medicines and in larger amounts than, say, supermarkets. The pharmacist may need to ask the purchaser a few questions before allowing specific medicine to be sold.

- ✔ **POM (Prescription Only Medicines):** Have to be prescribed and can't be bought over-the-counter.

- ✔ **CD (Controlled Drugs):** Prescription-only medicines. Controlled drugs are medically controlled under the misuse of drugs legislation (Misuse of Drugs Act, 1971). Examples include morphine, pethidine and methadone.

Distinguishing between generic and proprietary drugs names

Pharmaceutical companies patent their (new invention drugs) for up to 20 years from being deemed safe after undergoing clinical trials. This is when they make their medicine available and sell it under their brand name. For example: ibuprofen is a generic name for a medicine, whereas Nurofen or Hedex are the brand versions. Dangers arise in medications containing paracetamol, due to the addition of this drug in other medications, such as Night Nurse used to relieve the symptoms of chills or cold- and flu-like symptoms. Confused? Read on!

- ✔ **Generic medicines:** Use the chemical, officially approved or non-proprietary name of the drug. For example, salbutamol (albuterol) is used for asthma and other conditions associated with reversible airway obstruction.
- ✔ **Proprietary medicines:** Use the brand or trade name. For example, salbutamol is trade-marked as Ventolin.

Looking at Types of Medicine Administration

Medicines are presented to healthcare staff in many different forms and administered by various routes on and in the body, due to their variable modes of action.

For any drug to be effective, you have to administer it via the most suitable route, such as absorbed through the skin, bronchi or gastrointestinal tract and distributed to the site of action, usually via the circulation. The medication is then metabolised or broken down in order to be removed or excreted from the body – though some drugs may be eliminated without being metabolised.

In this section I discuss the different ways of getting the medication into the body and how they work.

Understanding how much of a drug actually works: Bioavailability

Medics need to consider the bioavailability when calculating dosages for non-intravenous routes of drug administration such as morphine (see Chapter 20).

Bioavailability is the proportion of the administered drug that reaches the systemic circulation and refers to the amount of drug available for distribution to the intended site of action. For example:

- ✔ Drugs administered by the intravenous route are considered to have 100 per cent bioavailability.

- ✔ Drugs administered via the oral route tend to have a decreased bioavailability. They're usually prescribed at higher doses than parenterally administered (injected) drugs, because not all the drug will be absorbed (oral drugs can be degraded by gastric acidity). Clinical relevance may then detect that your very nauseous patient would be better off having his antiemetic administered by injection, rather than by oral administration. Other non-injectable applications include oral, rectal, transdermal and sublingual.

The bioavailability of a drug can be affected by other factors such as:

- ✔ The patient's age, sex, genetic type and whether he has any malabsorption disorders or previous gastrointestinal surgery.

- ✔ How the drug is absorbed. Rapid absorption occurs if the drug is dissolved in aqueous solutions for intramuscular or subcutaneous injections. Delayed absorption occurs if the drug is injected as an oily solution, salt or polymer solution.

Bioavailability links with other terminology used in drug administration such as:

- ✔ **Pharmacodynamics:** What the drug does to the body. The interaction of the drug within the cell to produce biochemical or physiological changes in the body.

- ✔ **Pharmacokinetics:** The handling of the drug in the body, meaning:

  - • How the drug is absorbed in the body.

  - • How the drug is distributed around the body.

  - • How the drug is excreted or eliminated from the body.

- ✔ **Systemic medications:** Medications that refer to the whole body (check out the next section).

- ✔ **Topical medications:** Medications that refer usually to one site (see the later 'Applying externally: Topical medicines' section).

Working internally: Systemic medicines

Systemic medicines are drugs that affect the entire body and not just a single body part or organ. Table 6-1 shows some examples.

Table 6-1	Examples of Systemic Medicines
Systemic Medicines	**What Are They?**
Oral medicines – Solid dose	Tablets and capsules
	Soluble/dispersible/Effervescent tablets
	Lozenges
	Enteric coated tablets
	Sustained release tablets and capsules
Oral medicines – Liquid dose	Solutions
	Syrups
	Suspensions
	Emulsions
Rectal medicines	Medications for rectal administration (unsurprisingly)
Parenteral medicines (injected)	Intradermal
	Subcutaneous
	Intravenous
	Intramuscular
	Intra-articular
	Depot injections (see the nearby sidebar 'Injecting some explanations of parenteral medicines' for details)
Buccal	Dissolve between the cheek and gum
Sublingual	Placed under the tongue (get into bloodstream quicker)

Injecting some explanations of parenteral medicines

Parenteral drug administration means any non-oral means of administration, but today tends to be interpreted as the 'injectables'.

✔ **Intradermal:** Usually refers to vaccines and local anaesthetic products.

✔ **Intra-articular:** Injections received in the articular space between the joints.

✔ **Intrathecal injections:** Injected into the spinal canal, such as for spinal anaesthesia, chemotherapy and pain management.

✔ **Depot injections:** Eliminate the need to take a medicine every day, because the drug is released over a period of days, weeks or months. Depot injections are mainly administered via the intramuscular injection route and include antipsychotic medication, birth control and hydroxocobalamin injections prescribed for pernicious anaemia.

Applying externally: Topical medicines

Topical medications are applied to the outside of the body and include transdermal patches – such as for Hormone Replacement Therapy (HRT) and nicotine patches – gels, lotions and potions. Check out Table 6-2 for a few examples.

Table 6-2	Topical Medicine Examples
Topical Medicines	*What Are They?*
Ear, ear and nasal medications	Drops and sprays
Creams and ointments	Creams tend to be water-based or oily in water emulsions, and have moderate moisturising tendencies. Ointments tend to be oil-based preparations – containing 80% oil to 20% water proportions. Ointments are usually very moisturising and good for dry skin conditions.

Topical Medicines	What Are They?
Inhalers	Relievers and preventers
Rectal medicines	Suppositories
	Creams, ointments and foams
	Enemas
Vaginal preparations	Pessaries
	Devices – can be plastic, silicon and so on; used to treat a variety of medical conditions

Topical medication also refers to appliances such as anti-embolic compression stockings and medicated dressings.

Medications take variable times to have an effect within the body. For example, a very ill patient may require the IV format of a drug, rather than its intramuscular or oral format due to its quicker mode of action. As a handy guide, Table 6-3 gives some times that equate to the route of administration in an adult.

Table 6-3	Speed of Drugs Taking Effect with Different Administration Routes
Route	Time Until Drug Effect
Oral ingestion	30–90 minutes
Sublingual	3–5 minutes
Inhalation	2–3 minutes
Transdermal	Variable – minutes to hours
Subcutaneous	15–30 minutes
Intramuscular	10–20 minutes
Intravenous	30–60 seconds
Rectal	5–30 minutes

Giving special consideration to children and the elderly

You need to take special care when administering medications to youngsters and older people.

Paediatrics

Within the healthcare environment, under-16s or 18s are classified according to age:

- ✔ **Pre-term newborn infants:** <37 weeks gestation
- ✔ **Neonates:** 0–27 days
- ✔ **Infants and toddlers:** 28 days to 24 months
- ✔ **Children:** 2–12 years
- ✔ **Adolescents:** 12–16 or 18 years

The special considerations are required when administering drugs to younger people for the following reasons:

- ✔ **Children have differences in oral absorption, distribution, metabolism and excretion according to age and compared to adults.** For example, young children may require a higher dose per kilogram of their weight than adults owing to their higher metabolic rate.
- ✔ **Children have increased total body water as a percentage of their total body weight.** This total body water volume decreases with increasing age. For example, neonates, with a higher total body water volume, require higher doses of water-soluble drugs.
- ✔ **Many medicines aren't specifically licensed for paediatric use.** They may have undergone only adult drug trials.

For these reasons, children's doses may be calculated from adult doses using age, body weight or body surface area, or by a combination of these factors.

If a child weighing 20 kilograms requires ampicillin every six hours, this medicine may be prescribed as '80 mg per kg per day' on the prescription chart. Knowing the patient's body weight, you can work out how much of the medication the child requires with this formula:

Weight (kg) × Dose = 20 kg × 80mg = 1,600 per day

1,600 ÷ 4 (6 hourly) = 400 mg per dose

The most reliable methods are those based on body surface area, using a *nomogram* (a graph that relates a person's height or length, weight and surface area). When you've measured the height and weight, you can obtain the body surface area (BSA) with the nomogram (Figure 6-2 shows a nomogram).

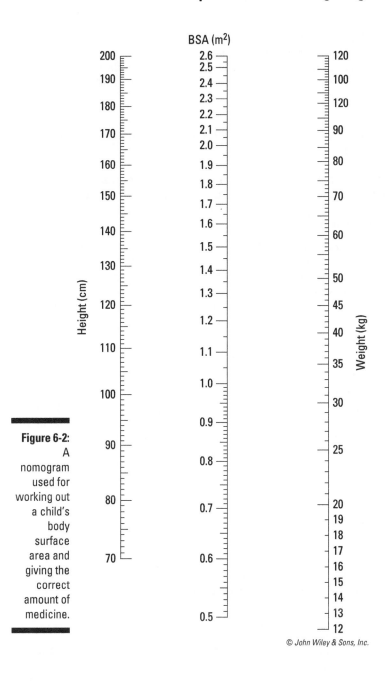

BSA (m²)

Height (cm)

Weight (kg)

Figure 6-2:
A nomogram used for working out a child's body surface area and giving the correct amount of medicine.

© John Wiley & Sons, Inc.

To find the BSA of an infant with a length 70 centimetres and a weight of 32 kilograms, place a ruler on the height scale of the nomogram graph at '70 cm' and across to the weight scale at '32 kg'. The straight edge then crosses the body surface area scale at 0.78 m², giving the child's BSA.

Geriatrics

The pharmacokinetics of drugs can be altered in the geriatric population in the following ways:

- ✔ **The elderly experience changes in oral absorption, distribution, metabolism and excretion with drugs as they age.** For example, the aging process can reduce gastrointestinal motility, which may affect the absorption of medications.

- ✔ **Older people have age-related reduction in kidney function, resulting in changes in eliminating certain medications.** For example, as renal function declines, drugs excreted via the renal system need to be adjusted. Also, due to metabolism, the half-life of drugs is increased as renal function is reduced. A drug's *half-life* is the amount of time it takes for a drug to lose half of its strength in blood plasma.

- ✔ **Liver metabolism can slow down, due to reduced hepatic blood flow, affecting the pharmacokinetics of a drug.** Therefore, you need to reduce hepatically cleared drugs in elderly patients.

- ✔ **The aging process can also have a significant effect on how the drug is distributed in the body.** For instance, as the body ages, muscle mass declines and the proportion of body fat increases, meaning that drugs that are fat soluble have a greater volume of distribution in an older person, compared to someone younger.

Working out drug dosages for the elderly, as with paediatrics, is often done using the following formula:

$$\text{Weight (kg)} \times \text{Dose}$$

Deciphering Doctors' Instructions on Prescription Charts

The *prescription chart* is a legal document, on which the doctor writes the medication prescribed, dose, route and times of administration, and any other directions. Some nurses are also drug prescribers.

You need to know your way around the prescription sheet, which is where this section comes in! Figure 6-3 shows a page from a typical prescription sheet.

RECOMMENDED TIMES OF ADMINISTRATION OF ANTIBIOTICS -		AFFIX PATIENT IDENTIFICATION LABEL	
		(If available)	

RECOMMENDED TIMES OF ADMINISTRATION OF ANTIBIOTICS -	
6 hourly	05.00 - 12.00 - 18.00 - 23.00
8 hourly	05.00 - 14.00 - 22.00
12 hourly	09.00 - 21.00

SURNAME (MR/MRS/MISS)	DATE OF BIRTH	UNIT NUMBER
FIRST NAMES	SEX	CONSULTANT
ADDRESS		

REGULAR PRESCRIPTIONS

	Date	Drug (Approved name-BLOCK CAPITALS)	Dose	Route	Times of Administration 6	12	18	23	Other Directions Duration	Doctor's Signature	Date	Pharm
1	TODAY	ERYTHROMYCIN	500MG	O	✓	✓	✓	✓		A Doctor		
2	TODAY	ASPIRIN (DISPERSIBLE)	300MG	O		✓			AFTER FOOD	A Doctor		
3	TODAY	TRAMADOL HYDROCHLORIDE	75MG	IV	✓	✓	✓	✓	GIVE OVER 28 MINS	A Doctor		
4	TODAY	PROPRANOLOL	80MG	O		✓	✓			A Doctor		
5	TODAY	HYDROXOCOBALAMIN	1MG	1M		✓			GIVE EVERY 3 MONTHS	A Doctor		
6	TODAY	KETOROLAC TROMETAMOL	35MG	IV		✓	✓		ADMINISTER OVER>15 SECONDS	A Doctor		
7												
8												
9												
10												
11												
12												
13												
14												
15												
16												

AS REQUIRED PRESCRIPTIONS

	Date	Drug (Approved name-BLOCK CAPITALS)	Dose	Route	Directions	Maximum Frequency	Doctor's Signature	Date	Pharm
1									
2									
3									
4									
5									
6									
7									
8									
9									
10									

Figure 6-3: One page of a prescription sheet.

© John Wiley & Sons, Inc.

Unless you know precisely what's written on the prescription chart, and what it means, seek direction/clarification from the doctor.

Knowing the abbreviations found on the prescription chart

Doctors often use abbreviations on their patients' prescription charts, even though many of these abbreviations shouldn't appear on the charts due to the possibility of errors. For example, 'IU' (to mean 'international units') written on the charts for insulin can be mistaken for '100'. Therefore, on the chart you can see acceptable and non-acceptable drug abbreviations.

To help you avoid coming a cropper, Table 6-4 lists abbreviations you may see on a prescription chart, including ones that can lead to errors and shouldn't be used.

Table 6-4	Abbreviations that Appear on Prescription Charts
Drug Abbreviation	*Full Name*
mcg or μg (shouldn't be used)	Micrograms (should be used)
IU (shouldn't be used)	International units (should be used)
PO	By mouth
mg	Milligram
IM	Intramuscular
g	Gram
IV	Intravenous
kg	Kilogram
SC	Subcutaneous
l	Litre
PR	Rectally
ml	Millilitre
NJ	Nasojejunal
TOP	Topically
PV	Vaginally
SL	Sublingual
Neb	By nebuliser

Drug Abbreviation	Full Name
OD (shouldn't be used)	Once daily (should be used)
BD (shouldn't be used)	Twice daily (should be used)
TDS (shouldn't be used)	Three times a day (should be used)
QDS (shouldn't be used)	Four times a day (should be used)
OM (shouldn't be used)	In the morning (should be used)
ON (shouldn't be used)	At night (should be used)
NG	Nasogastric
PEG	Percutaneous endoscopic gastrostomy
U	Units

Working around the (24-hour) clock

Within healthcare, the 24-hour clock, also known as the military clock, is the main system of time keeping. It runs on the principle of dividing the day into 24 hours, from midnight to midnight. For example, a doctor in a hospital setting doesn't write '6 a.m.' on the prescription chart, but '0600' hours (or '06:00').

Table 6-5 shows the 24-hour clock: try to become confident in using it to avoid any misunderstandings in drug administration.

Table 6-5	A 24-Hour-Clock Checklist
Time	24-Hour Clock
1 a.m.	0100 (01:00)
2 a.m.	0200 (02:00)
3 a.m.	0300 (03:00)
4 a.m.	0400 (04:00)
5 a.m.	0500 (05:00)
6 a.m.	0600 (06:00)
7 a.m.	0700 (07:00)
8 a.m.	0800 (08:00)
9 a.m.	0900 (09:00)

(continued)

Table 6-5 (continued)

Time	24-Hour Clock
10 a.m.	10:00
11 a.m.	11:00
12 noon	12:00
1 p.m.	13:00
2 p.m.	14:00
3 p.m.	15:00
4 p.m.	16:00
5 p.m.	17:00
6 p.m.	18:00
7 p.m.	19:00
8 p.m.	20:00
9 p.m.	21:00
10 p.m.	22:00
11 p.m.	23:00
12 midnight	24:00 or 00:00

1. Looking at the prescription chart in the earlier Figure 6-3, at what times has the erythromycin been prescribed (using the am/pm clock)?

   Answer: 6 a.m., 12 noon, 6 p.m., 11 p.m.

2. A prescription stating 12 hourly means that the drug should be given twice during the 24 hours, one stating 8 hourly means that the drug should be given three times during the 24 hours and one stating 6 hourly means that the drug should be given 4 times during the 24 hours.

   If the prescription before you states 4 hourly – how many times do you need to give the drug during the 24 hours?

   Answer: 24/4 = 6. Therefore, you give 6 times in 24 hours.

Telling IX from XI: Roman numerals

Doctors still, at times, use Roman numerals on the prescription chart, despite the practice not being encouraged. Therefore, you benefit from having a basic knowledge of this system and how it equates to ordinary numbers before kicking the doctor in the shins (only joking)!

Table 6-6 lists Roman numerals and their equivalent ordinary numbers.

Table 6-6	A Roman Numerals Conversion Checklist
Roman Numeral	*Ordinary Number*
I	1
II	2
III	3
IV	4
V	5
VI	6
VII	7
VIII	8
IX	9
X	10
L	50
C	100
D	500
M	1,000

Part II
Working Out Tablet and Liquid Dosages

Five great ways to maximise your skills when administering medications

- ✔ Apply the theory of calculations in the healthcare setting and become a competent practitioner.

- ✔ Use time-saving formulae when working out how many tablets or capsules to administer to the patient, according to the prescription.

- ✔ Memorise some easy-to-use formulae for when you're administering liquid medications, orally or by injection, to the patient.

- ✔ Master the advanced nursing calculations and become familiar with their use, such as when working out infant feeding requirements.

- ✔ Discover the make-up of so-called smart pills and increase your understanding of how they work.

web extras

To find out more about administering medication dosages, check out the free online article at www.dummies.com/extras/nursingcalculationsand ivtherapyuk.

In this part . . .

- ✔ Take physiological measurements to identify when drug intervention is required, such as when the patient's temperature deviates from the norm *(pyrexic)* and you give anti-pyrexic drugs.

- ✔ Understand the principles of injections and distinguish the different types, so that you can perform this skill correctly.

- ✔ Get to grips with diagnostic testing and how to perform these skills in venepuncture, to monitor blood levels such as urea and electrolytes.

- ✔ Spot adverse reactions, so that you can treat these potentially dangerous events effectively and efficiently.

Chapter 7

Measuring the Important Vital Signs

. . . .

In This Chapter

▶ Remembering the physiological measurements

▶ Seeing the warning signs

▶ Understanding fluid balance

. . . .

*I*n healthcare, you don't just need to be skilled at working out patients' drug dosages (see Chapters 2 to 6). A major part of a nurse's job involves monitoring and recording vital signs and fluid balance, and totting up these scores and running totals.

Clearly, these recordings need to be wholly accurate, because the measurements determine whether medical intervention is required. When plotting the vital signs on an observation chart, you need to know what this information means and be able to pick out the normal from the abnormal (a bit like watching *Britain's Got Talent*).

In this chapter, I talk you through physiological measurements, spotting where they indicate problems, and dealing with fluid balances.

Monitoring the Vital Signs: Physiological Measurements

Monitoring the vital signs links with the chapters in Part I of this book on the administration of drugs and calculations. For example, if the temperature rises you'd most probably consider giving the prescribed paracetamol at this point due to its antipyrexic properties.

In this section I cover breathing, pulse rate, temperature, blood, neurological observations and oxygen.

Respiratory rates – Don't hold your breath!

The *respiratory system* supplies the body with oxygen and removes the carbon dioxide through the rhythmic expansion and deflation of the lungs. Each respiration consists of an inhalation, exhalation and pause, before beginning the process again.

The act of breathing is called *ventilation,* and because this process is partially under the person's voluntary control, don't let the patient know that you're counting the rise and fall of her chest – the *respiratory rate.*

A change in a person's respiratory rate is a sensitive predictor of deterioration. By looking at the respiratory recordings on an observation chart, you can anticipate an adverse event, such as a cardiac arrest, four hours prior to its occurrence.

The respiratory rate consists of the number of breaths per minute. Normal respiratory rates vary according to age. Here are the accepted normal ranges:

- **Healthy adult:** 14–20 breaths per minute
- **Adolescent:** 18–22 breaths per minute
- **Children:** 22–28 breaths per minute
- **Infants:** 30 or more breaths per minute
- **Newborns:** 40 or more breaths per minute

A good respiratory assessment is measured over one full minute and includes monitoring of the following:

- **Rate of breathing:** Regular or irregular.
- **Depth:** Normal, shallow or deep.
- **Patient's colour:** Pink, flushed, *cyanosed* (blue tinge around mouth).
- **Sounds and ease of breathing:** Effortless, laboured, noisy, abnormal sounds.
- **Sputum production:** Sputum is an indication of a patient's wellbeing:
  - Bloody sputum may indicate bronchi inflammation, tuberculosis of the lung, lung abscess or embolism.
  - Rust coloured may indicate pneumococcal infection (pneumonia).
  - Purulent may indicate chronic lung disease.
  - Foamy white may indicate obstruction or oedema.
  - Frothy pink may indicate pulmonary oedema.

To help identify abnormal breathing patterns, you need to look out for the following (of course, these conditions all seem to have unnecessarily complex names!):

- ✔ **Dyspnoea:** Difficult, laboured breathing – shoulders are often raised, nostrils dilated and veins visible in the neck.

- ✔ **Cheyne-Stokes:** A gradual increase in the depth of respiration followed by a gradual decrease and then a period of no respiration *(apnoea)*. This syndrome is associated with end-of-life care.

- ✔ **Kussmaul's respirations:** An increased rate and depth of respiration with panting and long grunting exhalation – associated with lobar pneumonia.

- ✔ **Stertorous respirations:** Noisy respirations caused by secretions in the trachea or bronchi – may be due to partial airway obstruction.

- ✔ **Stridor:** A high-pitched noise heard on inhalation that's caused by laryngeal obstruction – a medical emergency.

- ✔ **Tachypnoea:** An abnormally rapid breathing rate.

Pulse rates: Keeping your finger on the pulse

To obtain a pulse rate, you gently feel *(palpate)* certain areas on the body, known as *pulse points*. At these points, an artery lies close to the surface of the body and you can feel and count the heart beats.

The radial artery in the wrist, due to its proximity, is the area of choice to determine the pulse rate. Figure 7-1 shows the sites of the major pulse points located on the body.

The pulse rate is more commonly known as the *heart rate* on observation charts.

As well as counting this rate over a one-minute time span, you also need to assess the regularity and volume: that is, monitor for any irregular pattern and strength of the beat.

An abnormal heart rhythm is known as an *arrhythmia,* which can be in two forms:

- ✔ **Tachycardia:** An abnormally fast heart rate (over 100 beats per minute in adults). This problem can be caused by raised body temperature, physical/emotional stress or heart disease, as well as by certain drugs.

✔ **Bradycardia:** An abnormally slow heart rate (less than 60 beats per minute). This problem can be caused by low body temperature and certain drugs. Fit athletes also tend to have low heart rates (like myself – I wish!).

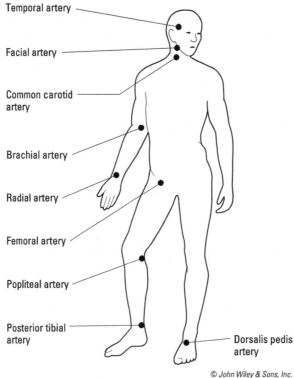

Temporal artery

Facial artery

Common carotid artery

Brachial artery

Radial artery

Femoral artery

Popliteal artery

Figure 7-1: Pulse points of the body.

Posterior tibial artery

Dorsalis pedis artery

© John Wiley & Sons, Inc.

REMEMBER

The normal heart rate (measured in beats per minute – bpm) varies according to age:

✔ **Newborn:** 120–160 bpm

✔ **1–12 months:** 80–140 bpm

✔ **1–2 years:** 80–130 bpm

✔ **2–6 years:** 75–120 bpm

✔ **6–12 years:** 75–110 bpm

✔ **Adolescent:** 60–100 bpm

✔ **Adult:** 60–100 bpm

Temperatures: Is it hot in here or is it just me?

Humans are usually able to maintain a constant core temperature (called *thermoregulation*) in spite of environmental changes (such as when the central heating's off in winter – brrrrr!).

But thermoregulation can go awry. Newborn and low-birth-weight babies, for example, don't have a robust thermoregulation system, and older people can also have an increased sensitivity to the cold.

People's body temperatures are classified into three groups:

- ✔ **Normothermia:** The normal body temperature of between 36–37.5 degrees Celsius.

- ✔ **Hyperthermia:** When the temperature is above the normal range. Causes of hyperthermia include infection, heat stroke, malignancy, stroke or central nervous system damage:

  - A temperature of 41 degrees Celsius can result in convulsions.

  - A temperature of 43 degrees Celsius renders life unsustainable.

- ✔ **Hypothermia:** When the temperature is below the normal range. Doctors sometimes induce hypothermia deliberately as a medical treatment, but it's more often caused by environmental exposure, medication or the exposure of internal organs during surgery. A temperature of 30 degrees Celsius is usually fatal to humans.

The body temperature is higher in the evening than in the morning, known as *the circadian rhythm*.

A rise in body temperature, above normothermia, is called *pyrexia* and is usually caused by a viral or bacterial infection. Antipyretic medication can be administered, such as paracetamol, to reduce the temperature. Pyrexia is often categorised as follows:

- ✔ **Low-grade pyrexia:** Above normal to 38 degrees Celsius.

- ✔ **Moderate to high-grade pyrexia:** 38–40 degrees Celsius.

- ✔ **Hyperpyrexia:** 40 degrees Celsius and above.

Usually, you measure a person's temperature in the following parts of the body:

✔ **Oral:** You place the thermometer in the *posterior sublingual pocket,* which is situated at the base of (and under) the tongue.

✔ **Axilla:** You place the thermometer in the centre of the armpit with the person's arm laid across her chest.

✔ **Ear:** You take the temperature in the ear with an infrared device called a tympanic membrane thermometer (see Figure 7-2). The *tympanic membrane* is a thin membrane, within the eardrum, that separates the external ear from the middle ear.

Insert the device snugly within the ear canal, which is covered with a clean disposable cover. Many hospitals have reconfigured tympanic thermometers to display the equivalent oral temperature reading. If not, the temperature in the ear is 0–3 to 0–6 degrees Celsius higher than an oral temperature.

✔ **Rectum:** You insert a special thermometer at least 4 centimetres into the anus of an adult and 2–3 centimetres in infants. Rectal temperature readings are usually about 1 degree Celsius higher than those taken in the ear.

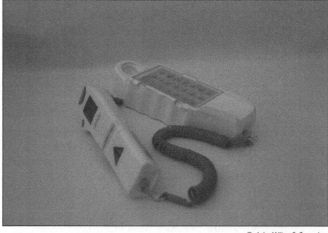

Figure 7-2: Tympanic thermometer for taking a patient's temperature in the ear.

© John Wiley & Sons, Inc.

You can take a child's temperature using *a tempo dot thermometer* (see Figure 7-3). This device is a 'smart-material' (*thermo-chromic* film), single-use plastic-coated strip, which has heat-sensitive dots that change colour to indicate temperature. You can place these strips across the child's forehead or in the mouth of an older child, making sure that she doesn't choke on it.

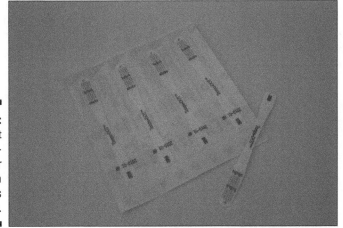

Figure 7-3:
Tempo dot thermometer for taking a child's temperature.

© John Wiley & Sons, Inc.

Blood pressures: Don't blow a gasket!

The blood pressure is the force with which the heart pushes blood through the blood vessels around the body. Blood pressure readings tend to increase due to many variables, including age, weight gain, stress and anxiety.

You combine two different readings to get the full blood pressure reading:

- ✔ **Systolic:** The reading you obtain when the ventricles in the heart contract, pushing the blood out under pressure. The systolic is the top or first number in a blood pressure reading.

- ✔ **Diastolic:** The reading you obtain when the ventricles relax, as the pressure decreases. The diastolic is the bottom or second number in a blood pressure reading.

A normal range for an adult is usually 100/60 to 140/90 mmHg (known as *normotension*): *mmHg* is the abbreviation for millimetres of mercury and is commonly used in medicine and other scientific fields to measure a manometric unit of pressure.

The following terms indicate abnormal blood pressure readings:

- ✔ **Hypotension:** Blood pressure that's lower than the normal range. It's generally treated, if causing problems, by lifestyle changes.

- ✔ **Hypertension:** Blood pressure that's higher than the normal range. It's more generally treated with medication, such as diuretics and/or anti-hypertensions. Lifestyle changes are also advised, such as reducing your salt intake to less than 6 grams per day and eating a healthy, low-fat diet. Losing weight, drinking less caffeine-rich drinks and alcohol, and being more physically active can also help reduce hypertension.

You can use many sorts of devices to take blood pressure, including automated blood pressure machines (automatic or oscillometric machines) and aneroid sphygmomanometers (used in conjunction with a stethoscope to hear the blood-pressure sounds). Figure 7-4 shows an aneroid sphygmomanometer (try and say that five times quickly!).

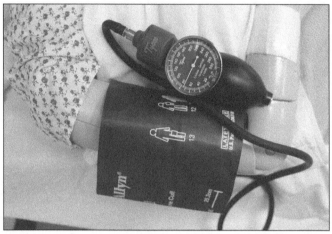

Figure 7-4: An aneroid sphygmomanometer taking a blood pressure reading.

© John Wiley & Sons, Inc.

Don't use automated blood pressure machines on patients with irregular heart rates, pre-eclampsia, certain vascular diseases or movement disorders such as Parkinsonian tremors.

Blood pressure cuffs need to cover 80 per cent of the circumference of the upper arm, or appropriate limb, because a poor fit renders an inaccurate reading. Also, the cuffs can get really tight (as you know if you've ever had a blood pressure reading taken), and so don't take blood pressure recordings on the limb of a patient who has an intravenous line: doing so can cause pain and damage to the line insertion site.

Neurological observations: Knowing the time, place and person

Many clinical areas use the Alert, Verbal, Pain, Unresponsive (AVPU) neurological response tool as a quick neurological assessment:

✔ **Alert:** Is the patient orientated to time, place and person? Use questions regarding the date/day and location, and asking the person to repeat her name.

 ✓ **Verbal:** Does the patient only respond to verbal intervention?

 ✓ **Pain:** Does the patient only respond to painful stimuli being inflicted?

 ✓ **Unresponsive:** Is the patient unresponsive?

Anything other than an 'A' (Alert) requires you to initiate a Glasgow Coma Scale (GCS) assessment (see Table 7-1).

Table 7-1	Quick Guide to the Glasgow Coma Score for Assessing a Patient's Level of Consciousness	
Eye Opening	*Best Motor Response*	*Best Verbal Response*
Spontaneous: 4	Obeys commands: 6	Orientated: 5
To speech: 3	Localises to pain: 5	Confused conversation: 4
To pain: 2	Withdraws to pain: 4	Inappropriate words (for example, random speech): 3
Nil: 1	Abnormal flexion to pain: 3	Incomprehensible sounds: 2
–	Extensor response: 2	Nil: 1
–	Nil: 1	–

You can conduct a full neurological assessment using the GCS, which looks at the patient's level of consciousness by assessing pupillary activity, motor function and verbal response. Each of these responses generates a score – the Glasgow Coma Score (which is used in conjunction with the vital signs observation chart): the lower the score, the lower the patient's conscious state.

The three measured responses have maximum scores – here's how to remember them:

 ✓ **Best motor response:** Generates a maximum score of 6. Remember with M (for motor) and 6 main motorways in UK = 6 motor responses.

 ✓ **Best verbal response:** Generates a maximum score of 5. Remember with 5 equals V (for verbal and the Roman numeral 5) = 5 verbal responses.

 ✓ **Eye opening:** Generates a maximum score of 4. Remember with 4 and eyes = four eyes = 4 eye-opening responses.

Table 7-2 shows how these numbers are generated more fully.

A painful stimuli is often performed using the *trapezium squeeze.* To perform this, use your thumb and two fingers to hold 5 centimetres of the adult trapezium muscle, where the neck and shoulder meet, and twist to observe for patient reaction. Ouch!

Table 7-2	Glasgow Coma Scores in More Detail
Grade of Response	*Information*
Best Motor Response	
6	The patient is able to carry out the simple things you ask, such as 'raise your arms above your head'.
5	The patient has a localising response to pain; that is, 'goes to' the pain site.
4	The patient is able to pull the limb away from the painful stimulus.
3	The painful stimuli causes abnormal flexion of the limbs.
2	The painful stimuli causes limb extension.
1	No response to pain.
Best Verbal Response	
5	Orientated to time, place and person.
4	Confused conversation – patient responds in conversational manner with some disorientation and confusion.
3	Inappropriate speech – random speech, with no conversational exchange.
2	Incomprehensible sounds – random noises/sounds.
1	No verbal response.
Best Eye-Opening Response	
4	Spontaneous eye opening.
3	Eye opening in response to speech or shouting.
2	Eye opening in response to a painful stimuli.
1	No eye opening.

Oxygen saturations: The champagne of life

Without oxygen, you die – bet that got your attention! *Oxygen saturation* is measured as a percentage by how much oxygen is attached to haemoglobin molecules and is being carried in the blood.

Oxygen can, however, be harmful under certain circumstances – causing *oxygen toxicity:*

✔ People with long-term conditions affecting the lungs or breathing muscles start to become accustomed to high carbon-dioxide levels, which then stop acting as a trigger within the body to breathe.

✔ These patients also become accustomed to lower oxygen levels, which now become the trigger to breathe.

✔ If these patients are given too much oxygen, the oxygen levels rise in their blood, causing them to lose their respiratory drive. Their respiratory rate gradually falls, carbon-dioxide levels rise and the patient can lose consciousness and die.

Oxygen saturations are routinely measured with a pulse-oximetry machine, a non-invasive device clipped on to a patient's finger, ear lobe or toe. The probe then emits red light, which passes through the tissue (for more, see the nearby sidebar 'Measuring oxygen saturations').

Target oxygen saturations, before intervention is required, are usually in the following regions:

✔ **94–98%:** Normal range for those aged under 70 years.

✔ **92–98%:** Normal range for those aged over 70 years.

A range of 88–92 per cent indicates that risk factors are present (for instance, chronic obstructive pulmonary disease; COPD).

Target saturations are prescribed on admission to hospital by the medical staff. Keeping within these targets is important, because a lack of oxygen means that bodily cells can't function normally, which can lead to cell damage, organ damage and patient death.

Measuring oxygen saturations

Pulse oximetry works on the principle that blood saturated with oxygen is a different colour than deoxygenated blood. The oxygen saturation is measured with a probe and the reading is displayed as a percentage on a screen.

The pulse oximetry recording can detect *hypoxia (SpO2)* – an inadequate or reduced tension of cellular oxygen, that is, tissue level. *Hypoxaemia (SaO2),* which is an abnormal deficiency of oxygen in arterial blood, can be detected only via arterial blood gases.

Pulse oximeters don't give accurate measurements if the patient is peripherally compromised or wearing nail varnish, because this interferes with the light source on the probe. Bright or fluorescent room lighting can also interfere with the probe's light transmission and patient movement such as rigours, shivering or Parkinsonian disorders can affect the pulse detections.

Identifying Deteriorating Patients

Gathering all the physiological observations and entering them on a chart isn't just a paper exercise: the results need to be assessed and acted on if required.

Acutely ill patients often exhibit abnormalities in their vital signs over a period of hours. These signs give healthcare professions time to intervene and offer prompt treatment, but only if they've monitored the trends on the chart and recognise that patients are deteriorating. This is known as *track and trigger* (tracking vital signs and triggering medical intervention).

The recommendation is that you then assess the patient's vital signs. A full patient assessment involves a systematic review – known as the A, B, C, D, E approach:

- ✔ **A = Airway:** Ask the patient to speak, which would indicate a patent airway in a conscious patient.

- ✔ **B = Breathing:** Count the respiratory rate and assess for any signs of respiratory distress and administer oxygen therapy if required.

- ✔ **C = Circulation:** Measure the BP and heart rate. Observe for signs of hypovolaemia – more about this in Chapter 14.

- ✔ **D = Disability:** This has four parts and involves assessing the patient's neurological status, blood glucose monitoring, looking at the patient's drug chart at the medicines she's taking and also at her urine output to review kidney status.

- ✔ **E = Exposure:** In order to examine a patient in her entirety, you may need to expose her, observing for signs of injury/bleeding and so on.

You can perform the A, B, C, D, E approach on all patients, not just those deteriorating.

Plotting the physical measurements on the observation chart

Document observations on the observation chart in black ink: they have to be clear and legible. If a manual observation has to be undertaken, as opposed to using machinery, also note this fact on the chart, usually by writing 'M' for manual. Lying and standing blood pressures should also be recorded on the chart and indicted with 'Ly' and 'St'. Apical heart beat deficits should also be noted to indicate 'apex' or 'radial' rates. Make all recordings with dots, rather than crosses or arrows.

To feel for an *apical pulse,* place a stethoscope on the chest wall adjacent to the apex cordi (first, find the fifth intercostal space). Perform this test if the radial pulse is abnormal or appears to skip a beat. Listen to the heartbeat, noting the rate and rhythm.

Spotting the danger signs: Early warning scores

Many healthcare areas use EWS (early warning score), MEWS (modified early warning score) or NEWS (national early warning score).

These systems use brightly coloured charts where each vital sign generates a score from 0 to 3. The following vital signs are observed (the earlier section 'Monitoring the Vital Signs: Physiological Measurements' has further explanations on each aspect):

- ✔ Respiratory rate (RR)
- ✔ Oxygen saturations
- ✔ Temperature
- ✔ Systolic blood pressure (BP)
- ✔ Pulse rate (often referred to as heart rate)
- ✔ Level of consciousness

A weighting score of 2 is also added for patients requiring supplemental oxygen therapy.

The higher the score, the farther the individual has moved away from the normal vital-sign parameter. The score then 'triggers' clinical action.

Table 7-3 shows an adaptation of the physiological parameters of the national early warning score (NEWS) system.

Table 7-3	National Early Warning Score System						
Physiological Parameters	*3*	*2*	*1*	*0*	*1*	*2*	*3*
Respiration rate	≤ 8		9–11	12–20		21–24	≥ 25
Oxygen saturations	≤ 91		94–95	≥ 96			
Any supplemental oxygen		Yes		No			
Temperature	≤ 35.0		35.1–36	36.1– 38.0	38.1– 39.0	≥ 39.1	
Systolic BP	≤ 90	91–100	101–110	111–219			≥ 220
Heart rate	≤ 40		41–50	51–90	91–110	111–130	≥ 131
Level of consciousness				A			V, P or U

Putting these parameters into practice, the two patients in Table 7-4 generate a NEWS score of 6 and 0; the table also shows how these scores are made up.

Table 7-4	Example of the NEWS System in Action	
	Patient 1	*Patient 2*
RR	21 = 2	15 = 0
Oxygen sats	96% = 0	98% = 0
Oxygen therapy	No = 0	No = 0
Temp	39.1 = 2	36.7 = 0
Systolic BP	180 = 0	130 = 0
Heart rate	120 = 2	80 = 0
Conscious level	Alert = 0	Alert = 0
TOTAL:	**6**	**0**

After you obtain the scores, you need to know what to do with them, apart from plotting them on a graph. Table 7-5 shows the clinical response to NEWS scores.

Table 7-5	Required Clinical Response to NEWS Scores	
NEWS Score	*Frequency of Monitoring*	*Clinical Response*
0	Minimum every 12 hours	Continue routine monitoring of NEWS with every set of observations.
Total 1–4 (a low score)	Minimum every 4–6 hours	Inform registered nurse, who must assess the patient. The registered nurse is to decide whether increased frequency of monitoring and/or escalation of clinical care is required.
Total ≥5 or 3 in one variable (a medium score)	Increased frequency to a minimum of once an hour	Registered nurse to inform urgently the medical team caring for the patient. Urgent assessment by a clinician with core competencies to assess acutely ill patients. Clinical care in an environment with monitoring facilities.
Total ≥7	Continuous monitoring of vital signs	Registered nurse immediately to inform the medical team caring for the patient – this team should be at least at speciality trainee level. Emergency assessment by a clinician team with critical care competencies, including practitioner(s) with advanced airway skills. Consider transfer of clinical care to a level-2 or 3 care facility: that is, a higher dependency or intensive care unit.

Finding Out about Fluid Charts

Accurately monitoring patients' fluid balances is crucial to their wellbeing. This section examines more closely what you need to know and why.

Checking fluid levels

The body works within narrow parameters and is always striving for balance *(homeostasis)*. Any water loss needs to be replaced so that the body's water volume remains constant:

- ✔ In males, the total body fluid constitutes approximately 60 per cent of the body weight.

- ✔ In females, total body fluid constitutes approximately 52 per cent of total body weight. (The rest is made up of 'sugar and spice and all things nice', as my mother used to say!)

Here's what can happen when a person's fluid levels aren't correct:

- ✔ **Hypovolaemia:** Too little fluid in the body due to diarrhoea, vomiting, sweating due to fever or blood loss.

- ✔ **Hypervolaemia:** Too much fluid, due to overinfusion of intravenous fluids, congestive cardiac failure, renal failure or hyperpyrexia (high body temperature, see the earlier section 'Temperature: Is it hot in here or is it just me?') brought about by taking the drug ecstasy and overhydration.

Maintaining the fluid balance

The volume of fluid lost by the body needs to be replaced by an equal amount of fluid – known as maintaining the *fluid balance*. To establish this total, all input and all output is recorded on the fluid chart like the sample in Figure 7-5. The output total is then subtracted from the input total, resulting in the balance. A greater input than output is recorded as a positive balance, but if input is less than output, a negative balance is recorded (but you'd look at trends over 2–3 days).

By adding up all the input in Figure 7-5, you can see that total fluid input is 2,050 millilitres. By adding up all the output, you find that it comes to 2,000 millilitres. Taking the output from the input reveals that this patient's 24-hour balance is 50 millilitres (positive).

Here are the daily inputs and outputs for an adult:

- ✔ **Typical daily intake includes:** 400 ml through metabolism, 500 ml from food and 1,500 ml from drinking. A total of 2,400 ml.

- ✔ **Typical daily output includes:** 400 ml through skin (due to perspiration), 400 ml through lungs (due to breathing), 1,500 ml from kidneys (urine) and 100 ml from intestine (faeces). A total of 2,400 ml.

24h Fluid Record	NO:
Date: _____ . _____ . _____	Surname: Forenames: Dob:
Previous Day's Balance: _____ml	Ward:

Time   Input Route (ml)   **Output Route (ml)**

Hour Ending	Oral	Enteral Tube	IV	Type	Running TOTAL	Urine	Gastric/Vomit	Faeces		Running TOTAL
08.00			1000 ml	N/S		550 ml				550
09.00										
10.00	150 ml				150					
11.00										
12.00	150 ml				300	300 ml				850
13.00										
14.00	150 ml				450		100 ml	150 ml		1100
15.00			1000 ml		1450	200 ml				1300
16.00										
17.00	150 ml				1600					
18.00	50 ml juice				1650	400				1700
19.00	250 ml water				1900					
20.00						300 ml				2000
21.00										
22.00	150 ml				2050					
23.00										
24.00										
01.00										
02.00										
03.00										
04.00										
05.00										
06.00										
07.00										
24h Total	1050		1000		2050 ml 24h Input	1750	100	150		2000 ml 24h Output

24h Balance = + 50 ml

Figure 7-5:
Typical fluid
chart.

What goes in – input

Fluids entered on the chart as *input* include

- ✔ Oral fluids
- ✔ Fluids administered via nasogastric tube
- ✔ Fluids administered intravenously
- ✔ Fluids administered subcutaneously

Fluid charts are rarely monitored as a one-off, but over a time limit of 2–3 days to get a full picture of the fluid balance.

What comes out – output

Fluids entered on the chart as *output* include

- ✔ Urine
- ✔ Vomit
- ✔ Wound drainage
- ✔ Liquid faeces
- ✔ *Insensible* loss (perspiration and water vapour excreted during respiration)

Insensible loss can account for 600–1,000 millilitres per 24 hours and therefore may need to be taken into account in acutely unwell individuals.

You can expect patients prescribed medication to increase their urinary output (known as *diuretics*) to have a negative balance.

Take a look at Table 7-6, which shows four patients' fluid balances.

Table 7-6	Fluid Balance Totals			
	Intake	*Output (ml)*	*Input Minus Output (ml)*	*Balance (ml)*
Patient 1				
	IV fluids = 1,000 ml			
	Oral fluids = 50 ml	Urine 1,070	1,050–1,070 = 480	–20

	Intake	*Output (ml)*	*Input Minus Output (ml)*	*Balance (ml)*
Patient 2				
	Orals fluids = 2 l	Urine = 500	2,000–500 = 1,500	+1,500
Patient 3				
	IV fluids = 1 l			
	Oral fluids = 500 ml	Urine = 750		
		Wound drain = 25		
		Vomit = 50	1,500–825 = 675	+675
Patient 4				
	Oral fluids = 750	Urine = 700	750–700 = 50	+50

Chapter 8

Sorting Out Medication Dosages

. . . .

In This Chapter

▶ Dosing up on formulae for giving pills

▶ Drip-feeding you information on liquid-dose calculations

▶ Titrating drugs appropriately and accurately

. . . .

*A*dministering medication is one of the most frequent nursing activities – and unfortunately one where mistakes occur. To decrease these errors, health professionals such as nurses and assistant practitioners require a robust understanding not only of the pharmacology of the medication, but also of the maths involved in administering the correct dosages.

This chapter helps you to gain confidence and competence when giving oral tablets and capsules and liquid doses of medication, as well as injectables.

Don't worry if you have to go over one or two of the questions a couple of times before the penny drops; you owe it to the patient to be slow and safe rather than rushing around like a whirling cartoon Tasmanian devil and getting the drug dosages wrong.

Figuring Out the Correct Oral Dose to Administer

Tablets and capsules are presented in variable strengths, and you'll be required to work out how many of these pills to administer to the patient.

 Before administering any medication, you need to know the contraindications, side effects and cautions. You find this information in the latest edition of the British National Formulary. You can also get info from pharmacists or your hospital's 'Drug Information' department, if it has one.

Perhaps the most important rule is: if you're unsure, ask.

Comparing oral drug administration methods: Bundles versus formulae

You can use one of two systems to work out how many pills to administer:

- ✓ **Bundles:** Breaking the dose down into smaller units.
- ✓ **Formulae:** Using an existing formula.

Bundles method

Your patient is prescribed 250 milligrams of a drug that's presented in a 1-gram format.

To use the bundle method, you need to break down the dose. Therefore, you convert both units to the same metric units, in this case the gram into milligrams:

- ✓ 1,000 mg = 1 whole tablet
- ✓ 500 mg = ½ tablet
- ✓ 250 mg = ¼ tablet

So to administer 250 milligrams, you give ¼ tablet.

This example is for illustrative purposes only. In real life you never break a tablet into quarters – you only ever cut a tablet in half, and only then if it's scored (with a line) and it's not a coated pill. You never break capsules in half (see Chapter 9 for more about smart pills).

If you do need to give someone a quarter-tablet amount, get the pharmacist to supply the drug in a different strength.

Formulae method

If you look at other nursing or medical books in relation to calculations and drug administration (though why you'd want to when you have this perfectly fabulous *For Dummies* book is beyond me!), you'll see many different expressions of the oral formulae for tablets and capsules.

Here's the formula I prefer to use:

$$\frac{\text{What you want}}{\text{What you've got}}$$

The sidebar 'Kittens and mittens and formulae' lists some more favourites.

Kittens and mittens and formulae

Here are a few of my favourite things . . .
I mean formulae:

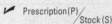 $\dfrac{\text{Strength required}}{\text{Stock strength}}$

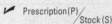 $\dfrac{\text{What you need}}{\text{What you have}}$

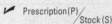 $\dfrac{\text{Prescription (P)}}{\text{Stock (S)}}$

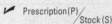 $\dfrac{\text{Amount of drug prescribed}}{\text{Amount of drug in each unit}}$

A nurse from overseas taught me this one:

$\dfrac{\text{What you desire*}}{\text{What we have in the cupboard}}$ (where the asterisk indicates a bar of chocolate!).

 Remember the dosage question? Your patient is prescribed 250 milligrams of a drug that's presented in a 1-gram format. Using my favourite formulae, you simply add the figures in their correct place in the formula:

$$\frac{\text{What you want}}{\text{What you've got}} = \frac{250\,\text{mg}}{1,000\,\text{mg}}$$

In words, 250 milligrams divided by 1,000 milligrams, which equals 0.25 (¼ tablet). (Again, for illustrative purposes only; you never break a tablet into quarters.)

 When using the formula, you need to make sure that both digits are in the same metric units (milligrams in this case).

 If you're a visual learner, picture a prescription chart when looking at the 'what you want' part of the formula and a bottle of pills when thinking about the 'what you've got part'. Also, good practice is to check whether the answer you come up with looks correct. For example, if your answer is 20 tablets, you know something has gone wrong with your calculations, because you'd never ask a patient to swallow 20 tablets in one go!

Formulae for more involved oral prescriptions

Formulae really come into their own when the questions get a more complicated!

 A patient has been prescribed 75 milligrams of atenolol (used to combat hypertension, angina, cardiac arrhythmias and migraine prophylaxis). The tablets are presented as 50 milligrams. How many tablets do you administer?

Using the $^{\text{What you want}}/_{\text{What you've got}}$ formula:

$^{75 \text{ mg}}/_{50 \text{ mg}}$ = 1.5 tablets = 1½ tablets

Table 8-1 shows more examples of using the formula method. If you need to brush up on your metric measurement abbreviations, flip to Chapter 2. Just remember: the 'what you want' part of the formula is what has been prescribed.

Table 8-1	Practice with Drug Calculations Oral Formulae		
Prescription	*How Drug Is Presented*	*Formula Using What-You-Want-What-You've-Got Formula*	*Answer*
750 mg ciprofoxacin	500 mg	$^{750 \text{ mg}}/_{500 \text{ mg}}$	1½ tablets
12.5 mg diazepam	5 mg	$^{12.5 \text{ mg}}/_{5 \text{ mg}}$	2½ tablets
225 mg ranitidine	150 mg	$^{225 \text{ mg}}/_{150 \text{ mg}}$	1½ tablets
125 micrograms digoxin	0.25 mg	$^{0.125 \text{ mg}}/_{0.25 \text{ mg}}$	½ tablet
60 mg codeine phosphate	30 mg	$^{60 \text{ mg}}/_{30 \text{ mg}}$	2 tablets
150 mg soluble aspirin	300 mg	$^{150 \text{ mg}}/_{300 \text{ mg}}$	½ tablet
750 mg penicillin	250 mg	$^{750 \text{ mg}}/_{250 \text{ mg}}$	3 tablets
7.5 mg bisoprolol fumarate	7.5 mg	$^{7.5 \text{ mg}}/_{7.5 \text{ mg}}$	1 tablet (formulae are designed to assist you, not to take away your ability to think: you don't need to use a formula here)
4 mg galantamine	12 mg	$^{4 \text{ mg}}/_{12 \text{ mg}}$	You can't administer a third of a tablet so you need to check how else this medication is presented
75 mg ascorbic acid	50 mg	$^{75 \text{ mg}}/_{50 \text{ mg}}$	1½ tablets

Knowing how many pills to administer

Tablets and pills can be available in many different strengths, and formats for that matter.

Always try to give the fewest number of pills, and in the best combination, as possible.

Warfarin comes in four dosages, as indicated on the bottle labels: 1, 2, 5 and 10 milligrams. Therefore, here's how you give the following dosages most efficiently:

- ✔ **To administer 4 mg of warfarin:** One 2-mg tablet plus one 2-mg tablet = 2 tablets.

- ✔ **To administer 9 mg of warfarin:** One 5-mg tablet plus one 2-mg tablet plus one 2-mg tablet = 3 tablets.

- ✔ **To administer 12 mg of warfarin:** One 10-mg tablet plus one 2-mg tablet = 2 tablets.

- ✔ **To administer 15 mg of warfarin:** One 10-mg tablet plus one 5-mg tablet = 2 tablets.

Working through some oral dose examples

In Table 8-2, I provide more examples of how a medicine is presented and the least amount of tablets/capsules to give to patients. Check out the table and get to grips with it all now!

Not all drug administration is easy – sometimes you need to think things through to find the best way of handing out the correct dose of medication. A great start is knowing for what medical conditions these drugs are given, and so check that the prescription is correct for the medical condition in the British National Formulary (www.bnf.org) – don't just take the prescriber's word for it.

Table 8-2	How Many Pills Do You Administer?		
Medicine	*Prescribed Dose and Reason for Prescription*	*How Drug Is Presented*	*Least Number of Pills to Administer*
Hyoscine butyl-bromide	15 mg three times daily for irritable bowel syndrome	10 mg	1½ tablets every 8 hours
Pyridoxine hydrochloride	75 mg for premenstrual syndrome	10 mg, 20 mg, 50 mg	50 mg + 20 mg + ½ 10-mg tablet = 2½ tablets
Ondansetron	16 mg one hour before anaesthesia	4 mg, 8 mg	8 mg + 8 mg = 2 tablets
Propranolol hydrochloride	Maintenance dose of 120 mg for angina	10 mg, 80 mg, 160 mg	80 mg + ½ 80-mg tablet = 1½ tablets
Carbamazepine	Initially 800 mg daily in two divided doses, as an adjunct in acute alcohol withdrawal (unlicensed)	100 mg, 200 mg, 400 mg	1 x 400 mg twice a day – 12 hourly = 1 tablet
Selegiline hydrochloride	10 mg in the morning for Parkinson's disease	5 mg, 10 mg	1 x 10-mg tablet = 1 tablet
Co-amoxiclav 250/125	One 250/125 strength tablet every 8 hours	No 250/125 strength tablets are in the drug cabinet, only 500/125	You can't use this strength, because cutting pill in half would present as 250/62.5
Erythromycin	500 mg every six hours for whooping cough for an 8-year-old child	250 mg	2 x 250 mg four times daily (every 6 hours) = 2 tablets
Danazol	800 mg daily in four divided doses	100 mg, 200mg	800 mg ÷ 4 = 200 mg per dose, 6 hourly = 1 tablet
Duloxetine	40 mg twice daily for moderate stress urinary incontinence	20 mg 40, mg	1 x 40 mg tablet, 12 hourly = 1 tablet
Lapatinib	1.25 g once daily for acute lymphoblastic leukaemia	250 mg	5 x 250 mg tablets per dose. Check to see whether dose available in a larger format = 5 tablets

Medicine	Prescribed Dose and Reason for Prescription	How Drug Is Presented	Least Number of Pills to Administer
Diclofenac sodium	150 mg daily in two divided doses for inflammation in rheumatic disease	25 mg, 50 mg	150 mg ÷ 2 = 75 mg per dose. 1 x 50 mg + 1 x 25 mg = 2 tablets

Calculating the Correct Liquid Dose

All injections need to be in liquid form, because pushing a dry tablet into someone's vein or muscle is difficult (please don't try)! Therefore, injectables need to be mixed in a transport medium (which isn't a Spiritualist riding around in a van!).

Not all liquid medications are for injection, of course: some are for ingestion, such as cough syrups, elixirs and linctuses. Liquid paracetamol for babies and children is also available. You work out the amount of medication to administer in the same way, however, using 'bundles' or a formula (check out the earlier section 'Comparing oral drug administration methods: Bundles versus formulae' for details on these two methods).

Bundles for liquids and injectable drugs

Gentamicin is dispensed as 80 milligrams in 2 millilitres. The prescription is to administer 60 milligrams of gentamicin. You break this amount down into smaller units, as follows:

- 80 mg in 2 ml
- 40 mg in 1 ml
- 20 mg in 0.5 ml

Therefore, to give 60 milligrams you use 1 millilitre (40 mg) plus 0.5 millilitre (20 mg) = 1.5 millilitres.

Formulae for liquid and injectable drugs

Here's how to use my favourite $^{\text{What you want}}/_{\text{What you've got}}$ formula (from the earlier section 'Comparing oral drug administration methods: Bundles versus formulae') for the same example.

The formula is the same as the one for tablets and capsules, except that because the medication is in liquid you have to add the volume:

$$\text{What you want}/\text{What you've got} \times \text{Volume}$$

As a result, the answer is always in millilitres, for example:

$$^{60\ mg}/_{80\ mg} \times 2\ ml = 1.5\ ml$$

Breaking this formula into bite-size chunks, you can see that the 'what you want' part is what's on the prescription form and the 'what you've got' part is what's on the packaging of the medication. You divide these two parts and then multiply by the volume.

Your patient is prescribed 8 milligrams of morphine IM. The stock ampoule label shows '10 mg/ml of Morphine Sulphate'.

To work out how much of the medication to draw up, use the $\text{What you want}/\text{What you've got}$ formula as follows:

$$^{8\ mg}/_{10\ mg} \times 1\ ml = 0.8\ ml$$

In words, 8 milligrams divided by 10 milligrams multiplied by 1 millilitre equals 0.8 millilitres.

Never lose sight of looking at the answer to see whether you think it looks right. For example, you know that 10 milligrams is presented in 1 millilitre, and so common sense tells you that the answer must be less than 1 millilitre: 0.8 millilitres seems right.

Many clinical areas expect two nurses to check medications for paediatrics or for injectables, to minimise mistakes.

Formulae for more involved liquid and injectable prescriptions

Here you get to put the what-you-want-what-you've-got formula through its paces when administering Oramorph.

You need to know that Oramorph (liquid) is presented in 100-, 300- and 500-millilitre bottles in strengths of 10 milligrams per 5 millilitres. They come in different sized bottles, but contain the same strength of drug at 10 milligrams per every 5 millilitres.

Your patient is prescribed 5 milligrams of liquid Oramorph from a 500-millilitre bottle. How much do you give?

The answer is:

$$^{5\ mg}\!\big/\!_{10\ mg} \times 5\ ml = 2.5\ ml$$

The doctor thinks again and prescribes the patient 5 milligrams of liquid Oramorph from a 100-millilitre bottle. How much do you give?

Answer:

$$^{5\ mg}\!\big/\!_{10\ mg} \times 5\ ml = 2.5\ ml$$

The doctor is vacillating (and driving you mad!). He now prescribes 7.5 milligrams of liquid Oramorph from a 500-millilitre bottle.

I hope you're catching on: this exercise shows that the bottle size is irrelevant. Whether you use a 100-millilitre bottle or a 500-millilitre one isn't a problem. The strength is what's important in your calculation, because the dose of the drug is fixed at 10 milligrams for every 5 millilitre. So how much do you give?

$$^{7.5\ mg}\!\big/\!_{10\ mg} \times 5\ ml = 3.75\ ml$$

After much deliberation, the infuriating doctor finally prescribes 12 milligrams of liquid Oramorph from a 500-millilitre bottle. How much do you give?

$$^{12\ mg}\!\big/\!_{10\ mg} \times 5\ ml = 6\ ml$$

Table 8-3 shows the side effects of Oramorph and the antidote to overdose.

Table 8-3	Side Effects and Antidotes to Oramorph Overdose
Side Effect	*Action/Information*
Constipation	Consider having *pro-re-nata* (as required) laxatives prescribed
Nausea and vomiting	Consider having antiemetics prescribed
Drowsiness	Often dose related and temporary – have medic review patient
Respiratory depression	Shouldn't occur if titrated correctly – have medic review patient
What is the antidote for an opiate overdose?	Naloxone – specifically designed to counteract the effects of the life-threatening depression of the central nervous system

Working through some liquid and injectable dose examples

Take a look at Table 8-4 to see how many millilitres of these drugs for injection you need to draw up for adult patients (Chapter 2 can help with any abbreviations you're unsure of).

Table 8-4	Worked Examples of Drug Doses for Injections		
Prescription	*How Drug Is Presented*	*Using What-You-Want-What-You've-Got × Volume Formula*	*Answer*
40 mg cortisone	50 mg in 2 ml	$^{40\ mg}\!/_{50\ mg} \times 2$ ml	1.6 ml
0.175 mg digoxin	500 micrograms in 2 ml	First change 0.175 mg into micrograms: $^{175\ micrograms}\!/_{500\ micrograms} \times 2$ ml	0.7 ml
270 mg erythromycin	300 mg in 10 ml	$^{270\ mg}\!/_{300\ mg} \times 10$ ml	9 ml
1750 units heparin	1,000 units in 1 ml	$^{1,750\ units}\!/_{1,000\ units} \times 1$ ml	1.75 ml
9 mg morphine	15 mg in 1 ml	$^{9\ mg}\!/_{15\ mg} \times 1$ ml	0.6 ml
125 micrograms digoxin	50 micrograms in 1 ml	$^{125\ micrograms}\!/_{50\ micrograms} \times 1$ ml	2.5 ml
9 mg gentamicin	20 mg in 2ml	$^{9\ mg}\!/_{20\ mg} \times 2$ ml	0.9 ml
250 mg flucloxacillin	1 gram in 10 ml	First change g into mg: $^{250\ mg}\!/_{1,000\ mg} \times 10$ ml	2.5 ml
85 mg pethidine	100 mg in 2 ml	$^{85\ mg}\!/_{100\ mg} \times 2$ ml	1.7 ml
0.6 mg naloxone	0.4 mg in 2 ml	$^{0.6\ mg}\!/_{0.4\ mg} \times 2$ ml	3 ml

Now check out Table 8-5 and see how many millilitres of these drugs for injection you need to draw up for some paediatric prescriptions.

Table 8-5	Worked Examples of Paediatric Drug Doses for Injections		
Prescription	*How Drug Is Presented*	*Using What-You-Want-What-You've-Got × Volume Formula*	*Answer*
Digoxin 18 micrograms	50 micrograms in 2 ml	$\frac{18 \text{ micrograms}}{50 \text{ micrograms}} \times 2$ ml	0.72 ml
Pethidine 20 mg	50 mg in 1 ml	$\frac{20 \text{ mg}}{50 \text{ mg}} \times 1$ ml	0.4 ml
Cephalothin 300 mg	500 mg in 2 ml	$\frac{300 \text{ mg}}{500 \text{ mg}} \times 2$ ml	1.2 ml
Flucloxacillin 400 mg	1 gram in 3 ml	First change grams in mg: $\frac{400 \text{ mg}}{1,000} \times 3$ ml	1.2 ml
Omnopon 16 mg	20 mg in 1 ml	$\frac{16 \text{ mg}}{20 \text{ mg}} \times 1$ ml	0.8 ml
Metoclopramide 4 mg	10 mg in 2 ml	$\frac{4 \text{ mg}}{10 \text{ mg}} \times 2$ ml	0.8 ml

Titrating Drugs According to Body Weight

Sometimes you're required to titrate drugs according to body weight (the patient's, not your own!).

This requirement is common with cytotoxic drugs used to treat cancers and when you're administering drugs to infants and children, as well as for patients in critical care and the elderly.

Checking out the formulae for titrating drugs

Here's the all-important formula to titrate drugs according to body weight:

Weight (kg) × Dose prescribed

The weight needs to be in kilograms for this formula. Therefore, you may need to convert stones and pounds into kilograms and even grams into kilograms for neonates.

Tables 8-6, 8-7 and 8-8 show, respectively, the conversions of kilograms to pounds, stones to kilograms and pounds to kilograms.

Here's a quick guide to the basic units:

- 1 kilogram = 2.2 pounds
- 1 stone = 6.35 kilograms
- 1 pound = 0.45 kilograms

You may find these weight conversion factors useful as well:

- **Stones to kilograms:** Multiply by 6.3503
- **Pounds to kilograms:** Multiply by 0.4536
- **Kilograms to stones:** Multiply by 0.1575

Table 8-6				Converting Kilograms to Pounds							
Kg	Pounds	Kg	Pounds	Kg	Pounds	Kg	Pounds	Kg	Pounds	Kg	Pounds
1	2.2	21	46.2	41	90.2	61	134.2	81	178.2	101	222.2
2	4.4	22	48.4	42	92.4	62	136.4	82	180.4	102	224.4
3	6.6	23	50.6	43	94.6	63	138.6	83	182.6	103	226.6
4	8.8	24	52.8	44	96.8	64	140.8	84	184.8	104	228.8
5	11.0	25	55.0	45	99.0	65	143.0	85	187.0	105	231.0
6	13.2	26	57.2	46	101.2	66	145.2	86	189.2	106	233.3
7	15.4	27	59.4	47	103.4	67	147.4	87	191.4	107	235.4
8	17.6	28	61.6	48	105.6	68	149.6	88	193.6	108	237.6
9	19.8	29	63.8	49	107.8	69	151.8	89	195.8	109	239.8
10	22.0	30	66.0	50	110.0	70	154.0	90	198.0	110	242.0
11	24.2	31	68.2	51	112.2	71	156.2	91	200.2	111	244.2
12	26.4	32	70.4	52	114.4	72	158.4	92	202.4	112	246.4
13	28.6	33	72.6	53	116.6	73	160.6	93	204.6	113	248.6
14	30.8	34	74.8	54	118.8	74	162.8	94	206.8	114	250.8
15	33.0	35	77.0	55	121.0	75	165.0	95	209.0	115	253.0
16	35.2	36	79.2	56	123.2	76	167.2	96	211.2	116	255.2
17	37.4	37	81.4	57	125.4	77	169.4	97	213.4	117	257.4
18	39.6	38	83.6	58	127.6	78	171.6	98	215.6	118	259.6
19	41.8	39	85.8	59	129.8	79	173.8	99	217.8	119	261.8
20	44.0	40	88.0	60	132.0	80	176.0	100	220.0	120	264.0

Table 8-7		Converting Stones to Kilograms	
Stones	*Kilograms*	*Stones*	*Kilograms*
1	6.35	15	95.25
2	12.7	16	101.6
3	19.05	17	107.95
4	25.4	18	114.3
5	31.75	19	120.65
6	38.1	20	127.0
7	44.45	21	133.35
8	50.8	22	139.7
9	57.15	23	146.05
10	63.5	24	152.4
11	69.85	25	158.75
12	76.2	26	165.1
13	82.55	27	171.45
14	88.9	28	177.8

Table 8-8	Converting Pounds to Kilograms
Pounds	*Kilograms*
1	0.45
2	0.9
3	1.35
4	1.8
5	2.25
6	2.7
7	3.15
8	3.6
9	4.05
10	4.5
11	4.95
12	5.4
13	5.85
14 (1 stone)	6.35

Paracetamol is prescribed as 10 mg/kg daily, to be administered every eight hours. How much do you give to a baby weighing 2.5 kilograms, daily and every eight hours?

You use the formula I give at the start of this section:

Weight (kg) × Dose prescribed = 2.5 kg × 10 mg = 25 mg daily

You then divide this answer by 3 to get the 8-hourly dose (because 24 hours contains 3 lots of 8) = 8.33 mg three times a day.

A child is prescribed 80 mg/kg/day of ampicillin, four doses per day. Calculate the size of a single dose if the child weighs 27 kilograms.

27 kg × 80 mg = 2,160 mg/day

Divide by 4 (four doses per day) = 540 mg for each dose.

Drum the following into your brain!

✔ Once daily = 24 hourly

✔ Twice daily = 12 hourly

✔ Three times daily = 8 hourly

✔ Four times daily = 6 hourly

Working through some titration dose examples

Table 8-9 shows how to titrate drug doses according to body weight.

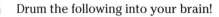

Table 8-9	Worked Examples of Titrated Drug Doses		
Prescription	*Patient's Weight*	*Formula: Weight (kg) × Dose Prescribed*	*Answer*
175 units/kg of tinzaparin per day	68 kg	68 kg × 175 units	11,900 units per day
30 mg/kg of streptomycin in three doses	48 kg	48 kg × 30 mg	1440 ÷ 3 = 480 mg
40 mg/kg erythromycin per day in four doses	12 kg child	12 kg × 40 mg	480 ÷ 4 = 120 mg

Prescription	Patient's Weight	Formula: Weight (kg) × Dose Prescribed	Answer
60 mg/kg chloramphenicol in four doses	44 kg	44 kg × 60 mg	2,640 ÷ 4 = 660 mg
2 mg/kg ranitidine per day	570 gram baby	Change grams into kg	0.57 kg x 2 mg
1.5 mg/kg enoxaparin	59 kg	59 kg × 1.5 mg	88.5 mg

Working out the dose according to body weight is only the first part of the question. Often, after titrating the medication according to the patient's body weight, you then use the $^{\text{What you want}}/_{\text{What you've got}}$ × volume formula (from the earlier 'Calculating the Correct Liquid Dose' section) to work out how much of the drug to draw out from the ampoule and administer to your patient.

Take a look at this example.

Solumedrol 2.5 mg/kg/hr is ordered for a child weighing 15 kilograms. Solumedrol is available as 125 mg/3 ml. How many milligrams of the drug does the patient require?

Weight (kg) × Dose = 15 × 2.5 = 37.5 mg

At how many ml/hr do you need to set the infusion pump?

$^{37.5}/_{125}$ × 3 ml = 0.9 ml

Try out this tester. Aggrastat at 18 mg in 132 ml is to be infused at 12 micrograms/kg/hr in a patient who weighs 14 kilograms. How many mg/hr of aggrastat does the patient require?

Here's the answer, but don't peek before having a go yourself:

14 × 12 micrograms = 168 micrograms

Change 168 micrograms into mg:

168 ÷ 1,000 = 0.168 mg

At what rate in ml/hr do you set the infusion pump?

$^{0.168\text{ mg}}/_{18\text{ mg}}$ × 132 ml/hr = 1.23 ml/hr

Chapter 9

Making Out the Make-Up of Pills

*B*efore administering any medication to patients, the nurse or other healthcare professional must understand the different types of drugs. In this chapter I describe how pills work in the body and how to interpret correctly a medication's information leaflet to avoid errors.

In addition, everything seems to be smart these days: smart phones, smart cars, smart energy meters and so on (perhaps scientists need to start work on people next!). Now you have smart pills. No, not high-IQ ones belonging to Mensa; these *smart pills* release the drug from the tablet over a period of time. I introduce you to a few types of such pills here as well.

Going through the System: How Drugs Work in the Body

Just as you need to develop the knowledge and skills to calculate drug dosages correctly, you also need to know about the medication you're administering to patients. In short, drug administration isn't a mechanical task – you need to know how the drug works within the body.

I cover the routes of drug administration in Chapter 6, such as oral, injection, creams and so on. You may want to check out that chapter before reading on.

One of the most common routes of drug administration is the oral route where the drug goes through the following stages:

1. **Dissolution:** The tablets/capsules break up into a soluble format in the presence of hydrochloric acid (in the stomach).

2. **Absorption:** This stage occurs in the small intestine, as the drug passes into the blood.

3. **Distribution:** The drug is released into the body via the bloodstream and passes through the liver.

4. **Metabolism:** The liver makes the drug inactive.

5. **Excretion:** The drug is passed out of the body.

Refer to Figure 9-1 for an illustration of where these different routes happen in the body. The following sections examine them more closely.

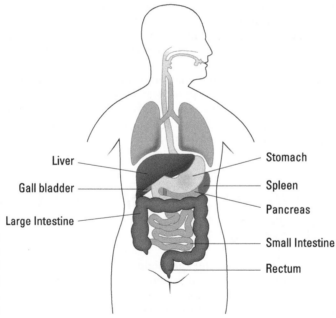

Figure 9-1:
Where the
body
absorbs
drugs.

Liver — Stomach
Gall bladder — Spleen
— Pancreas
Large Intestine — Small Intestine
— Rectum

© John Wiley & Sons, Inc.

Breaking down: Dissolution

Fortunately nothing to do with Henry VIII's breaking up of the monasteries; dissolution is the first stage where a pill taken orally is broken up in the stomach.

Medications administered via routes other than orally don't go through this dissolution process.

Knowledge of the process tells medical staff that, for example, paracetamol takes approximately 4–6 hours to dissolve. As a result, you can administer a second dose of paracetamol after 4–6 hours, with a maximum dose of 4 grams in 24 hours for adults.

You can't administer indigestion remedies at the same time of day as coated tablets (see the later 'Dressing up your pills: Medications with enteric coatings' section), because it causes premature dissolution, meaning that the drug starts dissolving before it reaches the systemic system, thereby making the pill less affective.

Being taken in: Absorption

Absorption is the movement of the drug from the administration site to circulating throughout the body's system. In oral drug administration, the following key factors determine the amount of the medication absorbed and the rate of absorption:

- ✔ Physical nature of the dosage form
- ✔ Presence of any food in the stomach
- ✔ Composition of the gastrointestinal contents
- ✔ Gastric or intestinal pH
- ✔ Mesenteric blood flow (blood flow to parts of the small intestine)
- ✔ Concurrent administration with other drugs

Drugs administered via the oral route tend not to have high bioavailability (see Chapter 6), and so are usually prescribed at higher doses than parentally administered (injected) drugs.

Spreading the feel-good factor: Distribution

Distribution is when the drug enters the bloodstream and is rapidly diluted and transported around the body. A number of important factors influence movement from the blood to the tissues of the body. One is the plasma proteins, which can bind many drugs. Only the unbound fraction of the drug is free to move from the bloodstream into tissues to exert a pharmacological effect.

The central nervous system is predominately surrounded by a specialised membrane, known as the *blood-brain barrier,* which is highly selective for lipid-soluble drugs. For example, penicillins diffuse well in body tissues and fluids, but in general penetrate poorly into the cerebrospinal fluid.

You can see an example of the blood-brain barrier in the treatment for Parkinson's disease – dopamine doesn't cross the blood-brain barrier and is therefore administered as a precursor. Levodopa is then administered and absorbed: it does cross the blood-brain barrier and is broken down to dopamine by the enzyme dopa decarboxylase. Bingo!

During pregnancy the placenta also provides a barrier between mother and foetus – some drugs cross it relatively easily (such as chlorpromazine and morphine) whereas others don't (such as suxamethonium chloride).

Make sure that you undertake the administration of medication during pregnancy with extreme caution, because physiological changes impact the pharmacokinetics of drugs during pregnancy, as shown in Table 9-1.

Table 9-1	**Pharmacokinetics of Drugs during Pregnancy**	
Stage	*Physiological Change*	*Effect*
Absorption	Gastrointestinal motility	Decreased
	Lung function	Increased
	Skin blood circulation	Increased
Distribution	Plasma volume	Increased
	Body water	Increased
	Plasma protein	Decreased
	Fat deposit	Increased
Metabolism	Liver activity	Increased
Excretion	Glomerular (renal) filtration	Increased

Soluble/effervescent medications work faster in the body because they bypass the dissolution process.

Converting drugs: Metabolism

Metabolism, simply put, is the chemical processes that occur within the cells of a living organism in order to maintain life. Drugs dissolve in gastric fluid and in order to diffuse across membranes they must be lipid-soluble. The higher the solubility in lipids, the more rapidly the drug diffuses into the tissues.

The main site of drug metabolism is the liver, but other tissues may also metabolise drugs, such as the following:

- ✔ Lungs
- ✔ Kidneys
- ✔ Blood
- ✔ Intestine

Eliminating waste: Excretion

The kidneys excrete most drugs. The rate of excretion varies greatly – some drugs are excreted within the hour and others take days or even weeks.

Individuals with renal impairment may excrete certain drugs more slowly, which has important consequences if the usual dose isn't reduced – plasma levels of the drug will rise, producing possible toxic effects.

Looking at Patient Information Leaflets

All medicines have a *patient information leaflet (PIL)* giving instructions on how to take or administer the medicine, listing all ingredients and detailing side effects. So you need to consult a PIL before giving a pill!

All these leaflets have the same basic layout and sections. As an example, I take a look now at one of these PILs in detail, in this case for a drug prescribed for breast cancer: exemestane 25 milligram coated tablets.

Examining a PIL

All PILs identify the drug in general and then move on to be more specific.

The information leaflet for exemestane starts by telling you that this drug is called Aromasin (the brand name) and that it belongs to a group of medicines known as aromatase inhibitors. These drugs interfere with a substance called aromatase, which is needed to make the female hormone oestrogen. The leaflet goes on to say that reducing the oestrogen levels in the body is a way of treating breast cancer.

The PIL then goes into more detail about what the drug is used for. The next section of the leaflet has advice about 'Before you take Aromasin' and 'Take special care with Aromasin', advising that this drug may lead to a loss of the mineral content of bones, which can decrease their strength.

The leaflet also informs that Aromasin shouldn't be taken at the same time as hormone replacement therapy and that a doctor needs to be informed if the following drugs are being taken, advising caution:

- Rifampicin (an antibiotic)

- Carbamazepine or phenytoin (anticonvulsants used to treat epilepsy)

- St John's wort herbal remedy

All PILs generally have sections on pregnancy and breast-feeding, driving, using machinery and important information about some of the ingredients and sugar intolerances. In addition, sections provide information on 'How to take [Aromasin]' and depending on whether the drug contains any substances related to these factors, what to do if you forget to take the drug or take more than you should. Other sections include 'How to store [Aromasin]' and what the drug contains and looks like in the pack.

Thinking about side effects

All drugs can cause unwanted side effects and interactions. By far the largest section in a PIL is the 'Possible side effects' one. Here are the four most important factors that predispose drug interactions:

- **Age:** Physiological changes occur as people grow older, which can affect the interaction of drugs. Liver metabolism, kidney function, nerve transmission and the functioning of bone marrow all decrease with age.

- **Polypharmacy:** The more drugs an individual takes, the more chance that some are going to interact.

- **Genetic factors:** Genes synthesise enzymes that metabolise drugs. Some genotype variations decrease or increase the activity of these enzymes.

- **Hepatic or renal diseases:** Drugs that are metabolised in the liver and/or eliminated by the kidneys may be altered if these organs aren't functioning correctly.

The Aromasin PIL's sections itemise the following side effects:

- **Very common side effects:**
  - Difficulty sleeping
  - Headache

- Hot flushes

- Feeling sick

- Increased sweating

- Muscle and joint pain

- Tiredness

✓ **Common side effects:**

- Loss of appetite

- Depression

- Dizziness

- Carpal tunnel syndrome

- Stomach ache, vomiting, constipation, indigestion, diarrhoea

- Skin rash, hair loss

- Thinning of bones

- Pain, swollen hands and feet

✓ **Uncommon side effects:**

- Drowsiness

- Muscle weakness

- Inflammation of the liver – hepatitis may occur

Getting to Know some Smart Drugs

I look at three types of smart pills in this section:

✓ **'Co' pills:** Feature two active ingredients.

✓ **Modified-release pills:** Have coatings to release their active ingredients over set times.

✓ **Enteric-coated pills:** Have specialised coatings to protect the stomach on their way to the circulatory system, or to protect the drug from the stomach acid, in order to release the drug into the intestines and so on.

Cuddling up together: 'Co' pills

Some medications contain two active ingredients combined together. This section looks at some of these pills/capsules, which you can identify by the 'co-' prefix written on the drug packaging. The drug name has a set of numbers after it (such as '2.5/20' or '8/500') that relate to the doses of the active ingredients within the medication. Table 9-2 lists eight examples of 'co' drugs.

Table 9-2	Eight Common 'Co' Drugs	
Drug Name	**What It Is**	**Active Ingredients**
Co-amilofruse 2.5/20	Potassium-sparing diuretic with other diuretic	Amiloride hydrochloride 2.5 mg, furosemide 20 mg
Co-amilozide 2.5/25	Potassium-sparing diuretic with other diuretic	Amiloride hydrochloride 2.5 mg, hydrochlorothiazide 25 mg
Co-amoxiclav 250/125	Penicillin	Amoxicillin 250 mg, clavulanic acid 125 mg
Co-beneldopa 125	Dopaminergic drug used in Parkinson's disease	Benserazide 25 mg, levodopa 100 mg
Co-careldopa 10/100	Dopaminergic drug used in Parkinson's disease	Carbidopa 10 mg, levodopa 100 mg
Co-codamol 8/500	Analgesic; anti-pyrectic	Codeine phosphate 8 mg, paracetamol 500 mg
Co-codaprin 8/400	Analgesic; anti-pyrectic; anti-platelet	Codeine phosphate 8 mg, aspirin 400 mg
Co-dydramol 10/500	Analgesic; anti-pyrectic	Dihydrocodeine tartrate 10 mg, paracetamol 500 mg

Moving slowly: Modified-release medications

Modified-release tablets and capsules are medications designed to dissolve and release their active ingredients over a set period of time, allowing the drug to enter the bloodstream in a steadier and more controlled way. They also save patients from having to take their medication at more frequent intervals.

Patients with Parkinson's disease, for example, are often prescribed their medication in a modified release. Here are some examples of modified-release drugs:

✔ Co-beneldopa

✔ Co-careldopa

✔ Pramipexole

✔ Ropinirole

Many different types of modified-release medications exist, as indicated by different abbreviations. For example, you may see the abbreviations 'SR' on medication packaging, which indicates 'sustained release'.

Here are some of the different modified-release abbreviations you encounter in practice, depending on the drug manufacturer:

- **CD:** Controlled delivery
- **CR:** Controlled release
- **DR:** Delayed release
- **ER:** Extended release
- **IR:** Immediate release
- **LA:** Long-acting
- **MR:** Modified release
- **SA:** Sustained action (can also mean 'short-acting' in some health authorities/ NHS Trusts)
- **SR:** Sustained release
- **TR:** Timed release
- **XL:** Extended release
- **XR:** Extended release
- **XT:** Extended release

The following important considerations apply when you're administering modified-release medications to patients:

- Time-release medications don't work as intended if they're split in half, because the controlled release coating on the pill is breached on the cut side. Also, capsules spill out their microbeads/powder and negate the modified-release aspect of the medication.
- Modified-release medications need to be swallowed whole and not chewed.
- Pharmaceutical companies don't always supply a range of variable doses for time-release medications, and so dosages tend to be more restricted.
- Patients who've had colostomies or ileostomies require a review of their medication (modified release and otherwise) due to drugs mainly being absorbed through the intestine and the surgery potentially having an impact on this process. Drug dosages may require decreasing.

Dressing up your pills: Medications with enteric coatings

The stomach is an acid environment and can destroy medication. Therefore, tablets and capsules can be coated with an outer coating to protect them from the acidity, avoiding the medication being broken down before it has a chance to get into the system to work. The coating can be added to cope with this gastric acid and is formulated to be dissolved only in the more alkaline environment in the small intestine – are these pharmaceutical scientists clever or what! Now you know why they're called 'smart' pills.

Enteric-coated medications usually have the logical abbreviation 'EC' on the packaging of the medication.

The coating is used on medications that may have an irritant effect on the stomach, such as aspirin. Other enteric-coated drugs include the acid-activated 'azoles' (such as omeprazole, which is prescribed for ulcers, dyspeptic symptoms requiring NSAIDs, *helicobacter pylori* eradication, Zollinger-Ellison syndrome and gastro-oesophageal reflux disease), and the modified-release medications I discuss in the preceding section.

We're leaving: Get your coatings

Materials used for enteric coatings include the following, starting with the most common:

- Shellac (hydroxyaliphatic acids and alicyclic acids – a natural polymer)
- Fatty acids
- Waxes
- Plastics
- Plant fibres

Medications that may contain shellac, depending on the pharmaceutical company, include:

- Amoxicillin 500 mg
- Clindamycin hydrochloride 150 mg
- Fluoxetine hydrochloride 20 mg
- Gabapentin 300 mg
- Lithium carbonate 300 mg
- Omeprazole 20 mg
- Omeprazole delayed release 20 mg
- Temazepam 15 mg

Chapter 10

Keeping Up to Scratch on Injections

*R*eceiving injections can be a prickly subject for patients (groan!), and their nervousness can transmit itself to the person giving the injection. As a result, you can both end up feeling needled (last pun, I promise).

The fear that many patients feel about even the thought of an injection means that you need to be as assured and confident as possible. Fortunately, this chapter is riding to your rescue. Here I describe all the injection types, correct skin preparation and different injection methods you can employ, and some of the tools you use too.

Exploring the Different Types of Injections

Injections are sometimes referred to as *parenteral* drugs (for bonus points, note that oral ones are called *enteral*). The main types of injection are:

- **Intradermal:** Drug is injected into the dermis layer of the skin.

- **Subcutaneous:** Drug is injected into the fat layer between the skin and the muscle.

- **Intramuscular:** Drug is injected into a muscle.

I look at each type in this section. I also discuss depot and intrathecal injections, with just a quick mention of intravenous injection (I explore this technique/ skill more fully in Chapter 14). I also give a quick call-out to my friend and yours *intra-articular* for the sterling work this type of injection, into the joint, does to relieve inflammation and increase joint mobility with corticosteroids on patients.

You can draw up parenteral-route medications from a glass or plastic vial or an ampoule with a rubber stopper with a syringe and needle prior to the injection. You can pre-draw up some injectables in the syringe ready to go. Sometimes the drug comes as a powder and needs to be reconstituted with solution and shaken to dissolve before drawing up into a syringe.

Before you give any type of injection, you need to know what layer of tissue you're aiming for. The skin has three primary layers, as shown in Table 10-1.

Table 10-1	Three Primary Skin Layers
Primary Layer	*Working from the Top downwards into the Body*
Epidermis (five layers, listed from top to bottom layer)	Stratum Corneum –Top Layer
	Stratum Lucidum
	Stratum Granulosum
	Stratum Spinosum
	Stratum Germinativum – Bottom Layer
Dermis (two layers – under the epidermis)	Papillary layer
	Reticular layer
Subcutaneous	Adipose tissue (sometimes referred to as hypodermis layer)

To remember the layers of the epidermis, try this little verse: Corny Lucy's Granny Spins Germs, which is short for Corne, Luci, Gran, Spin, Germ!

Tackling intradermal injections

You administer an *intradermal* injection just under the epidermis layer of the skin. The site is used for vaccinations, local anaesthetics and for diagnostic purposes – such as allergy testing or tuberculin testing. The effect is therefore often local and not systemic (affecting the whole body). Here are the locations of these injections:

✔ Anterior aspect of the forearm (medial forearm area)

✔ Back of upper arm

✔ Upper back

✔ Upper chest (scapulae)

Intradermal injections are administered using needle gauge size 25G, and at an angle of 10–15 degrees, needle bevel uppermost (see the later section 'Sizing up injection needles' for more details). Volumes of 0.5 millilitres or less are generally used for this injection route.

You inject the medication slowly and a *wheal* (a small blob or blister) should appear at the tip of the needle site. If a wheal doesn't appear, you've administered the injection via the subcutaneous layer and you need to withdraw the needle slightly until a wheal does appear.

Scratching the surface: Injection sites for subcutaneous injections

You give *subcutaneous* (SC) injections into the fat layer, underneath the epidermis and dermis layers of the skin, instead of into muscle.

Medication given via this route has a slow and steady absorption and the added advantage that blood vessels and nerves are minimal in these areas. Therefore, you don't need to *aspirate* (pull the syringe plunger back) after the needle has been inserted to check whether you've pierced a blood vessel and the medication is going to go into one; this occurrence is rare. Up to 1–2 millilitres of liquid can be delivered by this route, in adults, using a 25G needle or specialist syringe (all-in-one devices).

Medications given by the subcutaneous route include the following:

✔ Heparin

✔ Insulin

✔ Morphine

Here are the sites for subcutaneous injections:

✔ Abdomen

✔ Buttocks

✔ Thighs

✔ Upper arms

Check out Figure 10-1, which shows these sites.

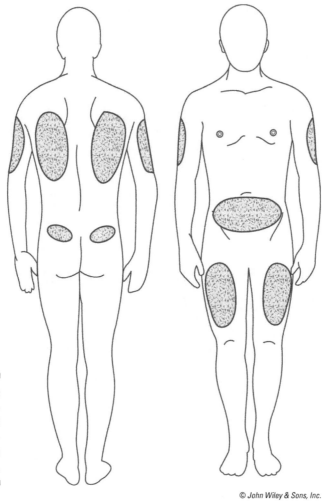

Figure 10-1:
Sites rec-
ommended
for subcuta-
neous
injections.

Showing your muscle: Injection sites for intramuscular injections

You administer *intramuscular* (IM) injections into the muscle below the subcutaneous layer, usually via one of four sites (see Table 10-2 for more details):

✔ Deltoid

✔ Dorsogluteal

✔ Vastus lateralis

✔ Ventrogluteal

Table 10-2	Four Injection Sites for Intramuscular Injections
Sites for IM Injection	*Information*
Deltoid	This site may not always be well-developed, and variable amounts of subcutaneous thickness exist between males and females. Procedure: Locate top of humerous bone and feel for greater tuberosity. Come below this site 2.5– 5 cm. Rotate arm to confirm site. 23G needles are suitable for most adults. Accommodates small quantities of drugs – maximum amount for adults: 0.5–1 ml, children and infants 0.5 ml.
Ventrogluteal (buttock)	This muscle is nestled in deep cavity far from bone, with no nearby nerves, veins or arteries. Procedure: Find the greater trochanter and then the top of the iliac crest. Inject halfway between these two, into the gluteus minimus. 21–23G needles are suitable for most adults. Accommodates 4 ml of drugs in adults, 2–2.5 ml in children and 1–1.25 ml in infants.
Dorsogluteal (buttock)	This muscle has a highly variable distance of skin to muscle (1–9 cm). This site also carries with it the danger of the needle hitting the sciatic nerve and superior gluteal arteries. Complications of this site also include fibrosis, nerve damage, abscess and necrosis. Procedure: Section the buttock into four imaginary panes. Inject into the upper outer quadrant of the top right pane. 21–23G needles are suitable for most adults. Accommodates 4 ml of drugs in adults, 2–2.5 ml in children and 1–1.25 ml in infants.
Vastus lateralis (thigh)	This site is free from major nerves and blood vessels and easily accessible for individuals who can't be turned. Procedure: Divide the thigh from hip to knee into thirds and inject into the bottom of the top third on the outer aspect of the thigh. 23G needle suitable for most adults. Accommodates 4 ml of drugs in adults, 2–2.5 ml in children and 1–1.25 ml in infants.

The injectable volume of medication administered by IM injection is variable, depending on the muscle bed. For example, in adults the deltoid can invariably only have 0.5–1 millilitres injected into this muscle, whereas the ventrogluteal, dorsogluteal and the vastus lateralis sites can have 4 millilitres injected.

Children have less muscle mass, however, and so administer half the adult volumes.

Types of medications given by intramuscular injection are many and varied, just a few being:

- ✔ Analgesics
- ✔ Antiemetics
- ✔ Narcotics
- ✔ Sedatives

Releasing the drug gradually with depot injections

You administer depot injections into muscle or adipose tissue beneath the skin to allow a deposit or *depot* of the drug into the chosen site. The drug is then released gradually into the systemic circulation over a period of time, once a week, once a month or longer.

This type of injection is often used in birth control, pernicious anaemia and antipsychotic medications, such as the following:

- ✔ **Flupenthixol decanoate:** Up to 400 mg every 2 to 4 weeks.
- ✔ **Fluphenazine decanoate:** Up to 100 milligrams (mg) every 2 to 5 weeks.
- ✔ **Haloperidol decanoate:** Up to 300 mg every 2 to 4 weeks.
- ✔ **Paliperidone:** Up to 150 mg every 4 weeks.
- ✔ **Pipoyhiazine palmitate:** Up to 200 mg every 4 weeks.
- ✔ **Risperidone:** Up to 50 mg every 2 weeks.

A depot injection takes away the worry and chore of having to remember to take medication on a daily basis.

Infusing the drug: Intravenous injections

The *intravenous* (IV) injection route (that is, one where the drug is injected directly into the vein) has many advantages over the other injection routes:

- ✔ It provides a rapid mode of action.
- ✔ It avoids the pain and irritation that can be caused by medications when administered by subcutaneous or intramuscular route.

✔ You can use it:

- For drugs that aren't absorbed by the gastrointestinal route.
- For drugs that become unstable in the presence of gastric juices and can be destroyed.
- Where patients can't tolerate fluid or nutrition via the oral route.

The intravenous route also offers control over the rate of administration of drugs.

I explore the disadvantages of using this route in Chapter 18, not least being the introduction of microbes, the inability to recall the drug and reverse its action, and needing to have an access port inserted, such as a *cannula* (a device inserted into the vein in order to act as a channel for the transport of medications directly into the bloodstream – the IV route; see Figure 10-2).

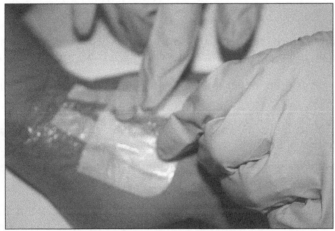

Figure 10-2: Inserting a cannula.

© *John Wiley & Sons, Inc.*

Methods of administering IV drugs include the following:

- ✔ **Continuous infusion:** Large amounts of fluid can be administered over a period of time, such as 1 litre of sodium chloride over 8 hours.

- ✔ **Intermittent infusion:** Smaller amounts of fluids can be administered, such as 50–250 millilitres of medication over a period of 20 minutes to 2 hours. Additional fluid or medication can be delivered through the primary line (therefore, two medications given simultaneously) – often referred to as a *piggyback* intravenous infusion.

- ✔ **Direct intermittent infusion:** Known as a bolus or push, the medication is injected directly into the access device (for example, the cannula) and usually over a short time span (3–10 minutes), depending on the drug.

Taking the spinal route: Intrathecal injections

This injection route is highly specialised, because the drug is administered to the cerebrospinal fluid (CSF) within the intrathecal space of the spinal column by lumber puncture or by specialist reservoir (Ommaya), which sits under the scalp and goes into a ventricle in the brain.

Although highly specialised, I mention this type of injection because nurses and other healthcare professionals may be involved in assisting medics to perform it.

This route is performed because some drugs have poor lipid solubility, or large molecules, and are unable to pass the blood-brain barrier. Molecules with a high electrical charge are also slowed. This reaction is a natural defence mechanism of the brain, protecting it from harm from 'foreign substances'.

Generally doses of medication for the intrathecal route are much smaller than those administered by intramuscular or intravenous injection.

Intrathecal drug administration is performed on patients in the following situations:

✔ Those with chronic spasticity due to injury, multiple sclerosis and cerebral palsy

✔ Those having chemotherapy treatment for lymphomatous meningitis

✔ For the management of cancer or neuropathic pain

✔ For antibiotic treatment adjuvant (to aid) a systemic antibiotic therapy in meningitis and other infections of the central nervous system

Lymphomatous meningitis is a complication of the most common type of blood cancer – lymphoma.

Cleaning Injection Sites

Cleaning the skin prior to administering subcutaneous or intramuscular injections is regarded as best practice in many hospitals.

Health centres may take the approach that skin disinfectant isn't always necessary, as long as the patient receiving the injection is physically clean and the person giving it maintains an aseptic approach.

In fact, patients receiving subcutaneous injections who repeatedly clean their skin with an alcohol swab may be harming themselves, because the alcohol may harden the skin and interfere with the insulin medication.

Always clean the skin of immunosuppressed patients to avoid introducing pathogens into the system, which can cause devastating effects.

When cleaning the skin, the site must be cleaned thoroughly with '2% Chlorhexidine in 70% Isopropyl alcohol' and left to dry for 30 seconds. 'Povidine Iodine 10%' must be used as an alternative if the patient is sensitive to Chlorhexidine.

The following skin cleaning products can be used for infants, depending on local policy and procedures:

- ✔ **0.05% Chlorhexidine:** For infants weighing less than 1.5 kilograms or aged less than 30 weeks.

- ✔ **0.5% Chlorhexidine:** For infants weighing more than 1.5 kilograms or aged more than 30 weeks.

Polishing up Your Injection Techniques

Clearly, developing a confident well-practised technique is important for nurses, because many patients are nervous about receiving injections and poor practice using the injection technique can present complications for them.

Here are just four of these complications, with tips and information to minimise these risks.

- ✔ **Abscesses:** If the medication in an aqueous medium is injected into fat, the drug isn't readily absorbed and a sterile abscess may form. This abscess may develop sepsis and become infected over time. To prevent abscesses always adhere to good practice and spend time identifying the correct injection layer using the right sized needle and try to alternate injection areas.

- ✔ **Infection:** To prevent infection, adhere to good hand hygiene and clean the injection site well, according to policy and procedures, and allow it to dry. Observe the injection site for swelling, redness or signs of cellulitis and report such problems immediately for treatment.

✔ **Haemorrhage:** To prevent IM haemorrhage, aspirate the syringe for 5–10 seconds to determine that the needle hasn't gone into a blood vessel. For SC injections, lift the adipose tissue away from the underlying muscle. Some patients are at more risk of developing a haematoma, namely those:

- On anticoagulation therapy

- With blood-clotting disorders

- With haemophilia

✔ **Pain:** To reduce pain, use a syringe and needle appropriate for patient, volume and body site. Insert the needle smoothly and quickly in a dart-like motion (though don't shout '180!' if all goes well) and administer the drug slowly. You can initiate distraction techniques, warning the patient to prepare for 'a sharp scratch'.

Bracing yourself to give SC and IM injections

Injections, such as SC and IMs, are given with the aid of syringe and needle (more about types of these later in this chapter in 'Tooling up to Inject: Equipment'). The key principle is to use the aseptic non-touch technique (ANTT), sometimes referred to as a *clean* technique, as opposed to an aseptic (or *sterile*) technique. I describe the ANTT in detail in Chapter 1.

Subcutaneous injection

The *subcutaneous layer* of the skin is beneath the dermis. The technique for administering an SC injection is by 'skin fold', because this technique is the only assurance that the injection goes into the subcutaneous layer (instead of as for an intramuscular injection and so having the wrong mode of drug action).

Using the thumb and index or middle finger, pinch up the dermis and subcutaneous tissue (up from the muscle tissue) – gently without causing a proper pinch! Create and maintain this skin fold throughout the injection, inserting an 8-millimetre insulin needle at a 90-degree angle.

The sites most commonly used for subcutaneous injections are the middle outer aspect of the upper arm, the middle anterior aspect of the thigh or the anterior abdominal wall just below the umbilicus, as shown in the earlier Figure 10-1.

Here's the procedure for SC injections:

1. **Explain procedure to the patient and gain consent.**

2. **Alcogel hands and put on gloves.**

3. **Check the drug, dose, patient, route, time and expiry date.**

4. **Draw up the medication using the aseptic non-touch technique (ANTT; see Chapter 1).**

5. **Expel any air and replace needle with a 25-gauge needle.**

6. **Clean the site if it's visibly dirty, the patient is elderly or immunocompromised, or it's near the site of an infection, and allow to dry.**

7. **Pinch a fold of skin to lift the subcutaneous tissue away from the underlying muscle.**

8. **Inject the medication gradually, into the chosen site, approximately at a rate of 1 millilitre per 10 seconds, at an angle of 90 degrees.**

9. **Withdraw the needle and dispose of promptly into a sharps bin.**

10. **Apply gauze or cotton wool to stop any bleeding.**

11. **Remove gloves and alcogel hands.**

12. **Document the administration of the drug.**

Intramuscular injections

Prior to administering an IM injection, conduct an assessment of the muscle mass of the injection site to establish needle size (see the later section 'Sizing up injection needles'). You administer these injections into the densest part of the muscle. The needle must penetrate the muscle but still allow a quarter of the needle to remain external to the skin.

If the patient is worrying about the thought of having an IM injection, employ the following techniques to reassure and minimise the pain:

- Use distraction prior to the injection.
- Position the patient so that he's comfortable.
- Help the patient to relax, so that the muscles are relaxed.
- Conduct an assessment prior to the injection: is the person needle phobic?
- Use ice or freezing spray to the injection site.
- Encourage the patient to ask questions so that he maintains some control over the situation.

The more tense the patient feels, the more pain he feels.

Here's the procedure for IM injections:

1. **Explain procedure to the patient and gain consent.**
2. **Alcogel hands and put on gloves.**
3. **Check the drug, dose, patient, route, time and expiry date.**
4. **Draw up the medication using the aseptic non-touch technique (check out Chapter 1).**
5. **Expel any air and replace needle with a 21–23-gauge needle, depending on depth required.**
6. **Clean the site if it's visibly dirty, the patient is elderly or immunocompromised, or if it's near the site of an infection, and allow to dry.**
7. **Stretch the skin (to reduce the sensitivity of the nerve endings to reduce pain) and insert the needle at a 90-degree angle.**
8. **Inject the medication gradually, into the chosen site, approximately at a rate of 1 ml per 10 seconds, at an angle of 90 degrees.**
9. **Withdraw the needle and dispose of promptly into a sharps bin.**
10. **Apply gauze or cotton wool to stop any bleeding.**
11. **Remove gloves and alcogel hands.**
12. **Document the administration of the drug.**

Keeping an eye on the curves: Meniscus effect

The *meniscus effect* is the curve in the upper surface of the medication in a syringe (oral or injectable) or pot used for liquid medication (see Figure 10-3). The effect is caused by the surface tension of the drug sticking to the sides of the container (a bit like a WAG sticking to a football player!). If you don't take account of the meniscus effect, you can end up giving an incorrect dose of medication.

The lowest level of the curve is the correct line to read. If using a medicine pot, always obtain this level by placing the pot on a flat surface and getting down to eye level to read the measurement.

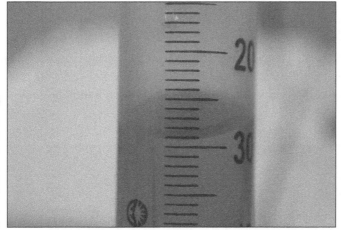

Figure 10-3: Meniscus effect in an oral syringe, showing a reading of 29 millilitres.

Tooling up to Inject: Equipment

When administering injections, picking the correct, fit-for-purpose, material is important. These sections can explain what you need to know.

Selecting the correct syringe

The syringe comprises a barrel to contain the liquid that's drawn up, with calibrations marked along the outer surface. A moveable plunger is inside the barrel with an end tip of different designs *(tip placement)* where the needle gets attached. Pulling this plunger back sucks fluid into the barrel, and pushing it in or forward expels this fluid.

Syringes come in a variety of calibrations, and as a general rule you shouldn't fill them to more than 75 per cent capacity, in order to allow for aspiration. Some syringes have a pre-attached needle (for example, ones used for insulin injection), and some come with a needle attached and are pre-filled with medication (for example, Clexane injections).

The next four figures show a selection of different syringes:

✔ Figure 10-4 shows a Luer Lock syringe, whereby the needle can be screwed onto the syringe for a secure lock.

✔ Figure 10-5 shows an eccentric Luer Slip syringe (one that wears its dressing gown and slippers to the supermarket), with the nozzle tip off-centre to allow closer application to the skin.

✔ Figure 10-6 shows a concentric Luer Slip syringe, used for all other applications, with the nozzle tip in the centre.

✔ Figure 10-7 shows an oral syringe, which shouldn't be confused with syringes used for injections.

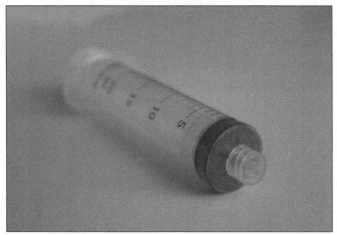

Figure 10-4:
A Luer Lock
syringe.

© John Wiley & Sons, Inc.

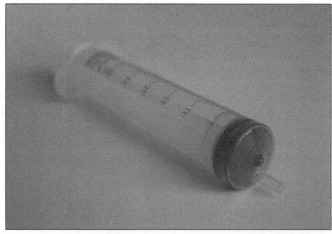

Figure 10-5:
An eccentric
Luer Slip
syringe.

© John Wiley & Sons, Inc.

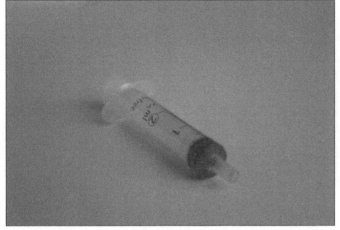

Figure 10-6:
A concentric
Luer Slip
syringe.

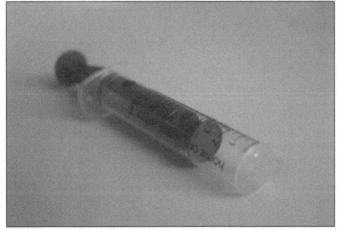

Figure 10-7:
An oral
syringe.

Sizing up injection needles

Needles are measured by their gauge size and length. They're colour coded, depending on the gauge size and manufacturer, and are presented in sizes from 18G to 30G, from largest to smallest. The larger the number gauge, the smaller the needle. Figure 10-8 shows three needles.

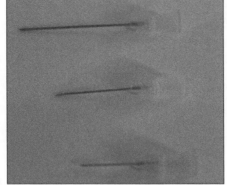

© John Wiley & Sons, Inc.

Figure 10-8:
Three injection needles, from top to bottom: 21G, 23G and 25G.

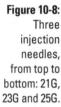

You need to conduct an assessment of the medication viscosity to be drawn up into the syringe, and for the actual administration of the drug, on each individual patient to assess for needle gauge size.

Also, assess the needle length size for each individual patient. For example, an injection into the buttocks depends on patient size:

- ✔ **21G, length 38 mm:** Suitable for most patients.
- ✔ **21G, length 50 mm:** Suitable for obese adults.
- ✔ **23G, length 25 mm:** May be suitable for particularly thin adults.

The gluteus muscles are likely to have atrophied in elderly, non-ambulant and emaciated patients, and males tend to carry more muscle bulk. If you don't conduct this assessment for needle length for intramuscular injection, most injections intended for the gluteal muscle are deposited into gluteal fat and not absorbed properly.

To assist in the patient assessment for needle length when administering intramuscular injections, you may want to calculate the Body Mass Index (BMI) of the patient, though BMI should be used *only as a guide*.

You obtain the BMI with the following formula:

BMI (in kg/m^2) = Weight (kg)/Height (m)^2

If a patient weighs 90.5 kilograms and is 1.82 metres in height:

$1.82 \times 1.82 = 3.3124$

$90.5/3.31 = 27.3$ BMI

According to the World Health Organisation classifications (see Chapter 12), this BMI makes the patient overweight. You need to take this fact into account when choosing the needle size when given the injection.

The bevel of the needle is the cut-out part of the needle: you administer injections with the bevel of the needle facing downwards (apart from intradermal injections, where the bevel faces uppermost). Figure 10-9 shows the bevel part of the needle (facing uppermost).

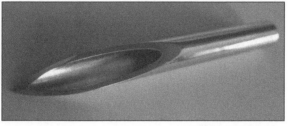

Figure 10-9:
Needle with bevel facing uppermost.

© *John Wiley & Sons, Inc.*

Wearing gloves

Adhering to strict hand hygiene when administering injections is vital. Use the aseptic non-touch technique (see Chapter 1), which is also known as the *clean* technique.

Wearing gloves when administering injections is considered best practice, because you're dealing with blood, which is a body fluid. Also, if you inadvertently sustain a needle-stick injury (see Chapter 18), some of the blood is wiped off the needle by the gloves, minimising the amount of patient's blood entering your system.

Chapter 11

Comprehending Diagnostic Blood Tests: Venepuncture

In This Chapter

▶ Introducing venepuncture basics

▶ Understanding blood tests and bottle types

*V*enepuncture is the procedure for obtaining blood samples for testing: you pierce the vein with a small needle to withdraw the sample. The samples of blood needed for testing are small, with even less required for children.

In this chapter I familiarise you with the skill of venepuncture (which sounds painful but isn't if done expertly!), help you identify normal and abnormal blood values, and guide you towards an understanding of blood tests.

Taking Blood to Test: Venepuncture

You carry out venepuncture for the following reasons:

✔ To obtain blood to rule out conditions

✔ To monitor levels of blood components

✔ To obtain blood for diagnosis

✔ To monitor blood levels

Table 11-1 shows the normal ranges of a selection of blood, medication and urine tests.

Anything outside these normal ranges invariably warrants medical intervention/treatment.

To brush up on your metric measurement abbreviations, flip to Chapter 2.

Table 11-1	Normal Values for Venepuncture Tests		
Test Name	*Units*	*Range Low*	*Range High*
Sodium	mmol/l	133	146
Potassium	mmol/l	3.5	5.3
Urea	mmol/l	2.5	7.8
Chloride	mmol/l	95	108
Bicarbonate	mmol/l	22	29
Phosphate	mmol/l	0.8	1.5
Magnesium	mmol/l	0.7	1.0
Osmolality	mmol/kg	275	295
Alkaline Phosphate (ALP)	u/l (unit/litre)	30	130
Creatine Kinase (CK)	u/l	40(M)/25(F)	320(M)/200(F) (M = Male, F = Female)
Bilirubin (total)	μmol/l	–	<21
Adjusted calcium	mmol/l	2.2	2.6
Urate	μmol/l	200(M)/140(F)	430(M)/360(F)
Carbamazepine	mg/l	4	12
Phenobaritone	mg/l	10	40
Phenytoin	mg/l	5	20
Lithium	mmol/l	0.4	1.0
24h urine urate	mmol/24h	1.5	4.5
24h urine phosphate	mmol/24h	15	50
24h urine magnesium	mmol/24h	2.4	6.5

Showing Some Bottle When Taking Blood

The sample bottles used for venepuncture have colour-coded bottle tops, which can vary according to manufacturer (see Figure 11-1). For example, a manufacturer may state that:

- ✓ Bottle sample 1 for clotting studies, needs to be a light blue top.

- ✓ Bottle sample 2 for Urea and Electrolytes (U&Es), need to be collected in a yellow top bottle.

- ✓ Bottle sample 3 for full blood counts, need to be collected in purple top bottles.

- ✓ Bottle sample 4 for cross matching, needs to collected in a pink top bottle.

✔ Bottle sample 5 for glucose needs, to be collected in grey top bottles.

✔ Bottle sample 6 for trace elements, need to be collected in dark blue top bottles.

I provide more information about these tests in this section.

If you have to collect multiple samples, you need to do so in a specific order depending of the Health Care trust. This *order of draw* is devised by pathology laboratories in each trust. The order is necessary because each bottle contains an additive, which may dribble out and contaminate the next sample.

This is why blood sample for specific tests can't be collected in any other tubes.

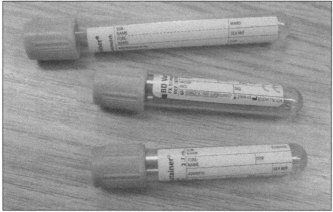

Figure 11-1:
Selection of venepuncture bottles for sample type.

© John Wiley & Sons, Inc.

Using bottle sample type 1

Depending on the manufacturer, you use this bottle sample type to collect for the following tests:

✔ Clotting studies

✔ D-Dimer (disseminated intravascular coagulation)

✔ Heparin monitoring

✔ INR

✔ Warfarin monitoring

These blood bottles contain the additive sodium citrate. Draw volume should be 2.7 millilitres per bottle, with less for children.

I describe some of the specific tests used in this bottle in this section.

Partial thromboplastin time

The activated partial thromboplastin time (aPTT) screening test measures the plasma coagulation factors of the intrinsic pathway, derived from the reagents used in the test to initiate the reaction: partial thromboplastin activator.

Simply put, the *intrinsic pathway* activates factor x to create the fibrin mesh to clot the blood.

The aPTT can be increased by:

- ✔ Deficiencies of plasma proteins specific to the intrinsic pathway
- ✔ Heparin
- ✔ Degradation products
- ✔ Pathological inhibitors
- ✔ Severely overdosed warfarin patients

Prothrombin

This test assesses the activity of the extrinsic pathway of blood coagulation; it can detect abnormalities in plasma coagulation. The time taken for the blood to clot when tissue factor and calcium is added is measured. The *extrinsic pathway* is an alternative of the clotting cascade. Its main function is to increase the activity of the intrinsic pathway.

Abnormalities are associated with the following:

- ✔ Anticoagulants
- ✔ Liver damage
- ✔ Vitamin K deficiency
- ✔ Warfarin overdoses

International Normalised Ratio (INR)

The INR test is a measurement of how long the blood takes to form a clot. The World Health Organisation introduced this test to provide a common basis for interpretation of prothrombin time (PT). International Normalised Ratio is calculated from the patient's PT ratio and a parameter called the International Sensitivity Index (ISI). Prothrombin time measurements are cheap and easy to perform, but the disadvantage is that large differences can result from laboratories. This is why the INR test was devised.

Putting bottle sample type 2 to the correct use

Depending on the manufacturer, you collect the following items using this bottle sample type:

- ✔ Amylase
- ✔ Antibiotic assays
- ✔ Calcium
- ✔ CRP (C-Reactive Proteins)
- ✔ Ferritin
- ✔ Folate
- ✔ Immunology
- ✔ Lipids
- ✔ Lithium
- ✔ LFT (Liver Function Tests)
- ✔ Magnesium
- ✔ Serology
- ✔ Serum electrophoresis
- ✔ Thyroid function test
- ✔ U&Es
- ✔ Vitamin B12

These blood bottles contain the additive SST II. Draw volume should be 5.0 millilitres per bottle, with less for children.

Check out some of the tests used in this section.

C-reactive proteins

This test has a similar function as the erythrocyte sedimentation rates (see the later section 'Erythrocyte sedimentation rates (ESR)') and is used to monitor the acute phase response of many infections.

In response to bacterial infection, trauma, tissue damage and inflammation, C-reactive protein levels rise dramatically.

Liver function

This process comprises of a number of tests to allow detection of liver disease, placing liver disease into a specific category and monitoring the progression of the disease. Liver function tests may also be conducted as a routine precaution after starting a new medication, to check that they aren't causing any liver damage as a side effect.

Urea and electrolytes

Urea is the waste product resulting from protein metabolism. Proteins are broken down by digestion into amino acids, which are then sent to the liver. The liver breaks them down further resulting in ammonia, which is toxic to the human body.

Urea measured from the blood serum sample allows monitoring of kidney and liver function.

High urea levels can indicate the following:

- Burns
- Congestive heart failure
- Renal disease
- Shock
- Urinary obstruction

Low urea levels can indicate the following:

- Liver failure
- Over-hydration
- Pregnancy
- Starvation

Electrolytes are minerals in your blood and other body fluids that carry an electric charge. Electrolytes include:

- Bicarbonate
- Chloride
- Creatinine
- Potassium
- Sodium

Severe dehydration causes a loss of water from the body tissues, often accompanied by an imbalance of sodium, potassium, chloride and other electrolytes. Prolonged dehydration can result in shock and damage to internal organs, particularly the brain, leading to confusion, coma and possible death. Quick – someone put up a drip!

Kidney function

The kidneys are used to filter waste materials from the blood and expel them as urine. They also play a part in controlling water and various minerals within the body. More specifically, they're critical to the production of the following:

- ✔ Hormones (to regulate the blood pressure)
- ✔ Red blood cells
- ✔ Vitamin D

Kidney function blood tests determine whether the kidneys are functioning correctly. They may also be carried out in patients with other conditions that can impact on the kidneys functioning and cause harm to the kidneys, such as those with hypertension and diabetes.

Symptoms of kidney problems can include

- ✔ Blood in the urine
- ✔ Difficulty beginning the process of urination
- ✔ Frequent urges to urinate
- ✔ High blood pressure
- ✔ Painful urination
- ✔ Swelling in the hands and feet due to fluid build up

Pancreatic function

The pancreas has a role in insulin production. This blood test can evaluate the function of the gall bladder and pancreas, because levels of the pancreatic enzymes amylase and lipase can be measured.

The pancreas also plays a vital role in digestion, and so any injury or injection to this organ can be extremely dangerous and requires urgent medical attention. Pancreatic cancer is one of the most dangerous forms of cancer, with a poor survival rate, and so early detection is vital.

Calcium levels

Calcium is the fifth most common element in the human body. Plasma calcium is necessary for maintaining a normal heart rhythm, the functioning of neurones, muscle contraction and is involved in the coagulation of blood.

Low plasma calcium levels *(hypocalcaemia)* can indicate

- ✔ Certain bone diseases
- ✔ Kidney damage
- ✔ Low calcium intake in the diet
- ✔ Low levels of parathyroid hormone
- ✔ Vitamin D deficiency

High plasma calcium levels *(hypercalcaemia)* can indicate

- ✔ Certain cancers
- ✔ High levels of calcium in the diet
- ✔ Increased levels of parathyroid hormone
- ✔ Overdose of Vitamin D

Cholesterol levels

Cholesterol is a major component of cell membranes; it's excreted in bile or metabolised in bile acids.

High levels of cholesterol in the blood can cause severe problems to the arterial and venous systems, building up on vessels causing inflammation, scarring and eventual blockage of the vessel.

Counting on bottle sample type 3

Depending on the manufacturer, these bottle sample types are used to collect for the following:

- ✔ Ammonia
- ✔ Full blood count
- ✔ Haemoglobin A1c
- ✔ Immunosuppressants
- ✔ Malaria screens
- ✔ Parathyroid hormone

🎯 Plasma viscosity

🎯 Sickle cell and thalassaemia

These blood bottles contain the additive ethylenediaminetetraacetic (EDTA; see the later 'Collecting blood with bottle sample type 4' section). Draw volume should be 4.0 millilitres per bottle, with less for children.

Read on to discover two of the tests used with this bottle.

Full blood counts

This blood test is one of the most common and is normally carried out as part of a routine check.

The haematology lab usually divides the *full blood count (FBC)* into five results:

🎯 **Differential blood count:** Identifies the concentrations of the five white blood cells:

- Basophils
- Eosinophils
- Lymphocytes
- Monocytes
- Neutrophils

🎯 **Haemoglobin concentration:** The oxygen-carrying component of erythrocytes. If this concentration is low, it usually indicates anaemia.

🎯 **Platelet count:** An integral part of the clotting system that basically plugs the hole where bleeding is present.

🎯 **Red blood cell count:** Erythrocytes are the most abundant cell type in the blood. By calculating their concentration, you can identify whether the patient is *anaemic* (low concentration) or *polycythaemic* (high concentration).

🎯 **White cell count:** Leukocytes form part of the body's defence against infections. They're normally found in low concentrations, unless an infection is present when the number increases.

Erythrocyte sedimentation rates (ESR)

This test measures the erythrocyte settling rate in anticoagulated blood, by measuring how fast the red blood cells, called erythrocytes, fall to the bottom of a thin tube. This test is used to determine how much inflammation is apparent within the body.

Tissue destruction and inflammatory conditions can cause a raised ESR and this result can be useful in assessing the degree of disease.

Collecting blood with bottle sample type 4

Depending on the manufacturer, you use this bottle sample type to collect transfusion samples:

- ✔ Antenatal
- ✔ Cross match
- ✔ Group and save

These blood bottles contain the additive EDTA (ethylenediaminetetraacetic – now you can see why it's abbreviated)! Draw volume should be 6.0 millilitres per bottle, with less for children.

The *cross match blood test*, sometimes known as a *compatibility test*, is a group of tests conducted to determine the most appropriate and compatible blood to be used as a transfusion, if one becomes required. Compatibility is performed by matching the intended recipient's blood with the donor's blood. This test is usually performed prior to undergoing a surgical procedure.

Pressing bottle sample type 5 into service

Depending on the manufacturer, you use this bottle sample type to collect the following:

- ✔ Ethanol
- ✔ Glucose
- ✔ Lactate

These blood bottles contain the additive fluoride oxalate. Draw volume should be 2.0 millilitres per bottle, with less for children.

Ethanol

This blood test detects blood alcohol levels. Alcohol is quickly absorbed into the blood and can be measured within minutes of having an alcoholic drink. The levels within the blood reach a peak after about an hour, depending how much food is in the stomach.

Blood alcohol levels are measured in milligrams per decility (mg/dl) with levels of 300–400 milligrams per decility (65.1–86.8 mmol/l) often proving fatal due to respiratory depression. One millimole of ethanol per litre of blood is equal to 4.61 milligrams of ethanol per 100 millitres of blood.

Glucose

Glucose is a simple monosaccharide produced as a result of the digestion process on starch/sucrose. The level of glucose in the body is highly regulated by the endocrine function of the pancreas.

Monitoring the blood glucose level allows medics to detect whether the patient has poor glucose level control. A high level *(hyperglycaemia)* may indicate diabetes.

Lactate

Lactate blood samples are collected for the investigation of *lactic acidosis* (low levels of oxygen in the body), which can be a presenting feature of a number of *inborn errors of metabolism*. These form a large class of genetic diseases involving congenital disorders of metabolism (mainly involving gene defects).

Related conditions of lactic disorders include the following:

- Acidosis
- Disorders of carbohydrate metabolism
- Glycogen storage disorders
- Inborn errors of metabolism
- Lactic acidosis
- Mitochondrial disease

Lactate blood samples also form part of the sepsis 6 – an initiative to reduce deaths from *sepsis* (blood poisoning). The sepsis 6 consists of putting three things into the body and taking three things out of the body within one hour of suspecting sepsis:

- **In:**
  - Oxygen therapy
  - Administer IV antibiotics
  - Give 20 ml/kg of IV fluids
- **Out:**
  - Take blood cultures
  - Measure levels
  - Lactate
  - Monitor urine output

Checking element levels with bottle sample type 6

You use this bottle sample type to collect the following (depending on the manufacturer):

- ✔ Aluminium
- ✔ Chromium
- ✔ Copper
- ✔ Fluoride
- ✔ Iodine
- ✔ Iron
- ✔ Manganese
- ✔ Selenium
- ✔ Zinc

These blood bottles contain trace element additives. Draw volume should be 6.0 millilitres per bottle, with less for children.

Aluminium

Aluminium levels may be increased in individuals on dialysis, or on aluminium antacid medications, and also in patients with renal failure and Alzheimer's disease.

Obtaining samples of blood to assess for aluminium levels may also be performed due to environmental factors and as an occupational-health blood test: that is, for people working in specific industrial sites.

Chromium

Chromium is a mineral that affects insulin carbohydrate fat and protein levels in the body. Increased chromium levels may occur if individuals are exposed to the substance by working in the leather tanning industry or steel manufacturing.

Copper

Copper is an essential mineral that the body incorporates into enzymes: excess and deficiencies of copper are rare.

Fluoride

Fluoride is an important mineral for the development of healthy teeth and bones. Over-exposure can result in respiratory problems, stomach pains and neurological problems.

Iodine

This test is rarely performed, but can be used to diagnose iodine deficiency and hypothyroidism.

Iron

Serum iron blood tests detect too high levels of iron in the blood, due to genetic conditions. They're also commonly requested when iron deficiency is suspected.

Manganese

This test is performed to measure manganese serum levels, because deficiency produces growth disorders, alters skeletal and cartilage formation, and impairs reproduction.

Selenium

Low doses of selenium are a requirement for good health. High concentrations are harmful and may cause

- ✔ Diarrhoea
- ✔ Nausea
- ✔ Vomiting

High oral doses can cause a condition known as *selenosis,* the major signs of which include the following:

- ✔ Hair loss
- ✔ Nail brittleness
- ✔ Neurological abnormalities (such as altered sensation/numbness in the extremities)

Zinc

Zinc is required in the body for the immune system and brain functioning. It also removes toxic metals from the brain, for example, copper, cadmium and mercury.

Zinc deficiency can contribute to many mental health symptoms. Here are some of the signs of zinc deficiency:

- ✔ Diarrhoea
- ✔ Hair loss
- ✔ Skin lesions
- ✔ Wasting of body tissues
- ✔ Worst case scenario: death

Clinical signs of zinc deficiency occur only when these levels become extremely low. Values less than 5μg/dl are particularly associated with loss of taste and smell, abdominal pain, diarrhoea, skin rash and loss of appetite.

Equally, too high levels of zinc in the body can be harmful by suppressing copper and iron absorption and other trace mineral blood tests.

Chapter 12

Using Advanced Formulae

*T*he calculations used in healthcare are becoming increasing complex, although that needn't necessarily equate to increased calculation errors. I'm a firm believer in using formulae to work out specifics, but to use a formula you have to know the whys and wherefores.

This chapter looks at some of the more advanced formulae that can assist you in your work, including body, organ and system calculations, and the special considerations involved when treating infants.

Dealing with Infants

Although staff sometimes call infants 'little people' affectionately, in the world of drug administration you can't consider them so. Things are more complicated than that. Here I discuss thinking about feeding requirements and growth expectations. Check out Chapter 6 for more on drug administration for paediatrics and neonates.

Calculating infant feeding requirements

Obviously, correctly preparing feeds for bottle-fed babies is important. A hungry baby usually cries between feeds and an overfed baby can experience diarrhoea and vomiting.

Infants need to receive 150–200 millilitres per kilogram body weight per 24 hours. Here's the formula for calculating feed:

Volume of feed = Amount of milk (ml)/Number of feeds in 24 hours × Weight of baby (kg)

Using that formula, calculate the volume of feed for a baby weighing 4.9 kilograms. He's fed 6 times every 24 hours. Remember that you need to calculate for the least (150 ml) and the most (200 ml) amounts.

Have a go yourself and then check out the answer:

Volume of feed = 150 ml/6 × 4.9 kg = 122.5 ml (least)

Volume of feed = 200 ml/6 × 4.9 kg = 163.3 ml (most)

Therefore, this baby requires between 122 and 163 millilitres in each feed.

Working out infant growth expectations

A newborn baby is expected to regain birth weight after two weeks and then gain the following:

✔ 200 grams per week until three months of age

✔ 150 grams per week for a further three months

✔ 100 grams per week until nine months of age

Three months is assumed to equal 13 weeks.

Imagine that you're required to calculate the expected weight of an infant aged 12 weeks whose birth weight was 3.2 kilograms. After two weeks, this infant weighs 3.2 kilograms again.

The answer is

12 − 2 = 10 weeks

At 200 g per week = 10 × 200 g = 2,000 g = 2 kg

Therefore, the expected weight = 3.2 kg + 2 kg = 5.2 kg at 12 weeks old.

Handling Body Calculations

Titrating drugs according to body weight is often performed when calculating doses for paediatrics and elderly patients and when administering cytotoxic drugs (for cancer); flip to Chapter 8 for more details. Another body calculation is working out the total body surface area (BSA) of the human body. As people grow in height and weight their skin surface area increases – this body surface area is measured in metres squared.

Delving into body surface area estimations

For neonates and children, using body surface area (BSA) estimates is more accurate than body weight when calculating drug dosages.

You calculate the dose required in the same way as weight (in kilograms) multiplied by dose, as I explain in Chapter 6, but you need to work out the surface area using a formula on a calculator.

Formula

The formula for working out the BSA (in square metres) is

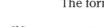

BSA (m²) = square root of (height (cm) × weight (kg)/3,600)

Here are a couple of examples that walk you through the steps.

Your first patient of the day is 1.70 metres tall and weighs 65 kilograms – you need to calculate her BSA:

1. **Convert metres into centimetres.**

   1 metre = 100 centimetres, and so 1.70 × 100 = 170 centimetres

2. **Multiple height by weight.**

   170 × 65 = 11,050

3. **Divide the result in step 2 (11,050) by 3,600.**

   3.0694

4. **Find the square root using a calculator.**

   1.75 metres squared

Next up, you need to find the BSA of a small child weighing 16.4 kilograms whose height is 100 centimetres. Therefore, in numbers, you calculate = 100 × 16.4/3,600:

1. **Multiple 100 by the weight 16.4.**

   1,640

2. **Divide 1,640 by 3,600.**

   0.456 (rounded up)

3. **Find the square root of 0.456 with your calculator.**

   0.675 m²

You can also find the BSA by using a nomogram. Pop to Chapter 6 where I describe the process and show you the graph.

The formula method and the nomogram method often give variable answers!

Average values as a guide

Table 12-1 shows useful average values for various parameters for when you're administering medications to children.

Only use these numbers if you can't find a specific dose, and always check them with the prescriber.

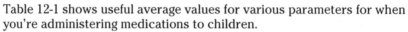

Table 12-1		Useful Approximate Values		
Age	*Weight (kg)*	*Height (cm)*	*Surface Area (m²)*	*Percentage of Adult Dose*
Newborn	3.4	50	0.23	12.5
1 month	4.2	55	0.26	14.5
2 months	4.4	51	0.28	15
3 months	5.6	59	0.32	18
4 months	6.5	62	0.36	20
6 months	7.7	67	0.4	22
8 months	8.5	72	0.44	25
1 year	10	76	0.47	28
18 months	11	90	0.53	30
3 years	14	94	0.62	33

Age	Weight (kg)	Height (cm)	Surface Area (m²)	Percentage of Adult Dose
5 years	18	108	0.73	40
7 years	23	120	0.88	50
10 years	30	142	1.09	60
12 years	37	145	1.25	75
14 years	45	150	1.38	80
16 years	58	168	1.65	90
Adult (male)	68	173	1.8	
Adult (female)	56	163	1.6	

Weighing in with the Body Mass Index

The Body Mass Index (BMI) is the most commonly used measurement of obesity, but it's also used to check that individuals are within a healthy range. A high BMI is associated with an increased risk of ill-health, such as cardiovascular disease.

The following is the formula for working out someone's BMI:

$$\text{BMI (kg/m}^2) = \text{Weight (kg)}/\text{Height (m)}^2$$

The World Health Organisation (WHO) classifies weight into BMI ranges (see Table 12-2).

Table 12-2	WHO Weight Classifications
Description	**BMI Range**
Normal	18.5–24.9
Overweight	25.0–29.9
Obesity Class I (moderate)	30.0–34.9
Obesity Class II (severe)	35.0–39.9
Obesity Class III (very severe)	> 40.0

Robert Simons is a student nurse. His height is 1.72 metres and he weighs 66 kilograms. Work out his BMI using the formula and his weight classification according to the WHO.

I hope you didn't peek before having a go yourself(!), but here's how you approach this problem, using the BMI formula:

$$1.72 \times 1.72 = 2.96$$

$$66 \text{ kg} \div 2.96 = 22.3 \text{ (rounded up)}$$

Therefore, Robert is classified as being in the normal BMI range.

A number of tables are available that do the work for you. Just by finding your weight and height, they show the band in which the BMI falls. But why make things simple? (No, don't write in with your answer to that!)

Making Organ and System Calculations

Some of the calculations you need to perform in the healthcare setting are in relation to the bodily organs and systems, such as cardiac output measurements, lung function and renal clearance measurements in order to establish how healthy, or poorly, your patients are. This section looks at the calculations and formulae used to gather this information.

Measuring cardiac output

Cardiac output is the amount of blood pumped by the heart's left ventricle (in millilitres) in one minute (expressed as ml/min). It's dependent on the amount of blood pumped out with each ventricle contraction – known as the *stroke volume* – and the heart rate (also known as the *pulse rate*). The stroke volume at rest in the standing position averages between 60 and 80 millilitres of blood in most adults.

Here are some of the factors that increase cardiac output:

✔ Anaemia

✔ Cirrhosis of the liver

✔ Pregnancy

✔ Severe infection

✔ Thiamine deficiency (beriberi)

To work out the cardiac output, you can use the following formula:

Cardiac output = Stroke volume × beats per min (pulse rate)

This formula is often expressed as CO = SV × P = ml/min

Given the stroke volume and pulse rates shown in the following list, I show the resulting cardiac outputs:

- **SV = 70 ml, P = 70 bpm:** CO = 70 × 70 = 4,900 ml/min
- **SV = 69 ml, P = 65 bpm:** CO = 69 × 65 = 4,485 ml/min
- **SV = 70 ml, P = 60 bpm:** CO = 70 × 60 = 4,200 ml/min
- **SV = 65 ml, P = 62 bpm:** CO = 65 × 62 = 4,030 ml/min

Assessing lung function

Pulmonary function tests are important tests used in the evaluation of respiratory health. They're conducted for the following reasons:

- To screen for the presence of obstructive and/or restrictive lung diseases.
- To evaluate the ability of a patient to be weaned off a ventilator.
- To assess the progression of lung disease and the effectiveness of treatment.
- To collect base line readings pre-surgery in order to determine the risk of respiratory complications post-surgery.

In the respiratory world, you need to know the following terms:

- **Vital capacity:** The amount of air that can be forcibly exhaled from the lungs after a full inhalation.
- **Forced vital capacity (FVC):** The amount of air forcibly exhaled from the lungs after taking the deepest breath possible.
- **Forced expiratory volume in one second (FEV$_1$):** The amount of air that can be forcibly exhaled from the lungs in the first second of a forced exhalation.

In order to assess the lung function, you use the following formula, which expresses it as a percentage:

The expired volume ratio = $(FEV_1 \times 100\%)/FVC$

Here's the process for calculating a person's total forced vital capacity when his FEV_1 is 4.5 litres and his FEV % is 90 per cent:

$$FEV_1\% = FEV_1 \times {}^{100\%}\!/_{FVC}$$
$$90\% = 4.5\,l \times {}^{100\%}\!/_{90} = 4.5\,l \times {}^{100}\!/_{FVC}$$
$$= 9 = 4.5\,l \times {}^{10}\!/_{FVC}$$
$$FVC = 9 = 45\,{}^{1}\!/_{FVC}$$
$$FVC = {}^{45}\!/_{9} = 5$$

Therefore, this person has a forced vital capacity of 5.0 litres.

Now, you need to calculate the forced expiratory volume $(FEV_1)\%$ for an individual with a FEV_1 of 4.2 litres and a FVC of 5.0 litres:

$$FEV_1\% = 4.2 \times 100\%/FVC\ 1$$
$$4.2/5.0 \times 100\%/1 = 84\%\ FEV_1$$

Checking out renal clearance measurements

Renal clearance refers to the ability of the kidneys to remove a given substance from the blood, in a given time. Here's the formula for calculating the renal clearance:

Renal clearance = (Urine × Volume)/Plasma

You can express this as $U \times V/P$.

Note that U = the concentration of the substance in the urine (mg/ml); P = the concentration of the substance in the plasma (mg/ml); and V = the volume of urine excreted (ml/min).

John Smith has the following recordings (in addition to all The Beatles albums!): U = 80 mg/ml, V = 120 ml/min and P = 55 mg/ml. Here's how you calculate John's renal clearance of creatinine:

$$80 \times 120/55 = 174.5\ ml/min$$

Looking at Additional Calculations

Here are a couple more formulae that may help you out from time to time.

Digging into dilutions

I explore solution concentrates in Chapter 5, but what if a prescribed solution isn't the same strength as the solution held in stock? In that case, you have to calculate the amount of stock solution and the volume of water to make up the prescribed solution.

Here's the formula for finding out this information:

Amount of Stock Required = Strength Required × Total Volume Required (ml)/Stock Strength

 Jeanette is to have a foot bathed in sterile normal saline. You need to prepare four litres of normal saline solution (0.9 percent). She has been prescribed 18 per cent of saline. You need to:

1. **Calculate the volume of stock that's needed when 18 per cent of saline is to be used.**

   $0.9\% \times 4\ l/18\% = 3{,}800$ ml is the volume of water

   $0.9/18 \times {}^{4{,}000}/_1$

   $9/180 \times {}^{4{,}000}/_1$

   9 goes into 9 = 1

   9 goes into 180 = 20 times = $^1/_{20} \times {}^{4{,}000}/_1$

   Remove 0 from 20 and 0 from 4,000 = $\frac{1}{2} \times {}^{400}/_1$

   2 goes in 2 = 1

   2 goes into 400 = 200 times = $^1/_1 \times 200 = 200$ ml of 18% saline

2. **Work out the volume of water to use:**

   ${}^{0.9\%}/_{18\%} \times 4\ l = 200$ ml

   4,000 ml minus 200 ml = 3,800 ml

   3,800 ml is the volume of water required.

Working out the energy requirements of the body

Energy calculations are generally performed by doctors and dieticians, but nurses can be asked to participate in the calculations when completing nutrition charts for patients.

Energy is measured in kilojoules (kJ). A calorie is a unit that indicates a food's energy value: 1 calorie is equal to 1,000 kilocalories (kcal) and 1 kcal = 4.2 kJ.

Got that? Great. The average person should derive his energy sources from the following:

- 15 per cent from protein
- 35 per cent from fat
- 50 per cent from carbohydrate

For more details, visit `http://www.nutrition.org.uk/Facts/energynut/energy.html`.

If a 35-year-old postman requires 3,000 kilocalories per day, how many of these 3,000 kilocalories should come from fat?

$$3,000 \times 35\% = 3,000 \times \frac{35}{100} = 1,050 \text{ kcal}$$

To convert this amount into kilojoules:

$$1,050 \times 4.2 = 4,410 \text{ kJ}$$

A keen jogger has an energy requirement of 250 kJ/kg of body weight per day. If she weighs 50 kilograms, how many kilocalories does she require in one day?

$$250 \times 50 = 12,500 \text{ kJ per day}$$

Converted in kilocalories = $12,500 \text{ kJ} \div 4.2 = 2,976 \text{ kcal per day}$

Here's another little puzzle to keep your grey cells ticking over.

A patient is on a strict low sodium diet totalling 2,400 calories per day. The dietician asks you what his estimated caloric intake is for the day.

Find the answer as follows:

- **Look at the nutrition chart:** You see that he ate only 50 per cent of his breakfast, lunch and tea.
- **Work out the answer by multiplying the desired intake of 2,400 calories by the percentage the patient consumed:** $2,400 \text{ kcal} \times 50\%$.

  Or more clearly: $2,400 \text{ kcal} \times 0.5 = 1,200 \text{ kcal}$ (the amount of calories the patient has consumed today)

Chapter 13

Monitoring Patients for Adverse Reactions

*A*dverse reactions are when a patient sustains an injury caused by taking a medicine (and not when your friends say that they don't like your new Saturday-night outfit!). In this chapter, however, I cover not only adverse reactions to medications, but also allergies to everything from wasps to wheat. Plus I describe the processes for dealing with a serious, life-threatening, anaphylactic shock.

So the next time a patient yells, 'Why are my lips swelling?', you know how to respond (and the answer isn't, 'Oh my! That looks awful. You must be devastated!').

Understanding Adverse Reactions

The most severe forms of allergic reactions tend to stem from environmental factors, dietary allergens and medication, such as to penicillin.

When you're administering medications via the intravenous (IV) route, the drug enters the body quickly and can be especially problematic when the body reacts to the drug badly.

Adverse reactions can be caused by many different means, however, not just medications, and so I give you an overview of adverse reactions in this section.

Healthcare professionals should not only be able to recognise and manage correctly when patients are experiencing adverse drug reactions (ADRS), but also when they're reacting to other triggers, such as latex or injected venom.

The most serious type of allergic reaction is full-blown anaphylaxis. Here I introduce you to anaphylaxis, anaphylactic shock, anaphylactoid and panic attacks:

- ✔ **Anaphylaxis:** A life-threatening type of allergic reaction that involves the airway, breathing and circulation and usually occurs rapidly.

- ✔ **Anaphylactic shock:** Anaphylaxis is also known as anaphylactic shock due to systemic vasodilation when due to symptoms of *myocardial depression* (a drop in blood pressure) causing hypotension and brady-cardia, which is a late feature, and often preceding a cardiac arrest (flip to Chapter 7).

- ✔ **Anaphylactoid:** Anaphylaxis is a whole body reaction to an *allergen,* a substance that can cause an allergic reaction. After being exposed to an allergen the body's immune system becomes sensitised to it. When the person is exposed to the allergen again, an allergic reaction can occur. Anaphylactoid is the name of the first exposure to the *antigen* (the substance that causes the immune system to produce antibodies against it).

- ✔ **Panic attacks:** May be confused with anaphylactic reaction. Individuals who've previously had anaphylaxis events may be prone to panic attacks if they believe that they've been re-exposed to an allergen.

Now for the technical bit: an *antibody* is a protein produced by the immune system in response to the presence of an allergen (the antigen causing the allergic reaction), which is in or on a foreign antigenic material. The immune system creates antibodies known as IgE.

The next time the allergen enters the body, it cross-links the IgE antibody bound to the mast cell (the white blood cell called leukocyte). This triggers the mast cell to degranulate, releasing histamine and other inflammatory mediators. The inflammatory mediators are now able to bind to receptors on target cells, which leads to symptoms of allergy.

Comparing allergies and anaphylaxis

Confusion sometimes arises over the difference between allergies and anaphylaxis. An *allergy* is a hypersensitivity of the immune system, for example:

- ✔ Asthma

- ✔ Allergic Rhinitis (hayfever)

- ✔ Eczema

Anaphylaxis is the most severe form of allergic reaction and is defined as 'a severe life-threatening generalised or systemic hypersensitivity reaction'.

Recognising anaphylaxis

True anaphylaxis involves the airway, breathing and the circulation, which is what makes this condition life-threatening. People often die from anaphylaxis because they don't obtain medical assistance quickly enough and go into anaphylactic shock. For instance, they may not ask for medical assistance because they don't recognise the symptoms of an anaphylactic reaction: the feeling of 'a lump in my throat' and a rasping husky voice, with tingling in the mouth and a feeling of dizziness.

Anaphylaxis is an exaggerated response of a previous sensitised individual to a *foreign antigenic* material: something the body sees as an invading protein, which it seeks to destroy. This means that the individual has had a previous exposure to this substance, the antigen, but may have no knowledge of the previous exposure – perhaps because it was so mild.

An anaphylactoid (the initial exposure to the antigen) needs no specific anti-body, because this occurs on the first exposure. Further exposures are now called anaphylaxis events.

Don't stand over an individual who has collapsed on the floor, semi-conscious, and wonder whether she's experiencing an anaphylactoid or anaphylaxis event – *both can be fatal!* They can both present with the same following symptoms:

- ✔ Laryngeal oedema
- ✔ Bronchospasm
- ✔ Hypotension

They both require the same treatment (see the later section 'Managing Anaphylaxis Events').

Triggering anaphylaxis by medication

Previously, doctors in hospitals gave the first dose of IV antibiotics and the nurse then administered the second or third doses.

This is no longer the case, because medics now know that the reaction is more likely to occur after the second or third dose of exposure to the foreign antigen. For this reason, nurses now administer first and subsequent doses of IV therapy, but should undertake anaphylaxis training.

Individuals at risk of a severe reaction, and who need to be particularly careful to avoid their problematic allergen, include the following:

✔ Those with asthma

✔ Those suffering from an infection

✔ Those who've exercised just before or just after coming into contact with the allergen

✔ Those suffering from emotional stress

✔ Those who've consumed alcohol

✔ Those who've been travelling abroad (think communicating in a foreign language)

The most severe reactions are likely to follow injections, especially those by the IV route. But that doesn't mean that administering medications via other routes can't cause the problem as well. Whichever route you use can cause a reaction, and possible anaphylaxis, because the allergen still enters the body and sets off a chemical cascade in response. So you need to be aware of the potential problem with routes, such as:

✔ Inhalation

✔ Intramuscular (IM) injection

✔ Oral

✔ Rectal

✔ Subcutaneous injection

✔ Topical

✔ Vaginal

Phylaxis is seldom used today, but the word means protection in Greek. Anaphylaxis therefore means the opposite: without protection.

Covering the causes of anaphylaxis

In this section, I describe the four most common causes for anaphylaxis: food, injected venom, medication and latex. Food is the most common trigger in children, but in adults drugs are most common.

Food

Up to ten recognised deaths occur from food allergy in the UK every year. Therefore, health professionals need to be aware of and recognise patient triggers.

Food triggers can include the following:

- ✔ Peanuts
- ✔ Tree nuts (walnuts, pecans, pistachios, cob nuts, cashews, almonds)
- ✔ Shellfish
- ✔ Fish
- ✔ Milk
- ✔ Pulses – lentils
- ✔ Sesame
- ✔ Soy
- ✔ Wheat
- ✔ Eggs
- ✔ Some fruit and vegetables (apples, pears, cherries, melon pumpkin, peas, beans, strawberries and tomatoes to name just a few – the list is endless)

Sometimes, the food ingredients can be 'hidden' in the foodstuff. For example, peanut oil is in many foods, such as bread and biscuits, or in factories handling nuts. Therefore, the foodstuffs can be contaminated. Also, food ingredients may be added to non-food products: for example, children's 'cradle cap' shampoo often contains peanuts (arachis oil) and many drug capsules have casings containing milk proteins, which affect people suffering from lactose intolerance.

Here are some more examples where food ingredients may be added:

- ✔ **Almond oil:** May be added to hair shampoos, bath and shower gels, and fabric softeners.
- ✔ **Avocado:** May be added to skin moisturisers.
- ✔ **Fruits:** May be added to skin products and lip balms.
- ✔ **Macadamia nuts:** May be added to hair-straightening balm.

Even commercially produced play dough can contain allergens – it's a minefield!

The advice is, of course, always to read the ingredients on packaging. Reading them may not be as easy as it sounds, however, because someone with a milk allergy may not be aware, when reading the ingredients on a product such as a condom, that casein is a milk protein. Vaccines may also contain small amounts of egg protein, which may not be suitable for those with egg allergies: even playing with egg boxes may trigger a reaction in those with severe allergies. Health professionals and those working with children must have knowledge of this information, because children often use egg boxes when crafting designs in the hospital setting with therapists.

For another problem, check out the nearby sidebar 'It's all Latin to me'.

Injected venom

The venom from bites and stings can trigger an anaphylaxis event in susceptible individuals. Here are a few examples:

- Ants
- Bees
- Hornets
- Wasps
- Yellow Jackets

Although individuals with allergies are told to avoid the problematic allergen, they may not easily be able to do so when going out into the big outdoors!

It's all Latin to me

Sometimes manufacturers list their produce ingredients in Latin, meaning that people reading the lists may not know that the item is the very thing that they're allergic to. Here are a few of these Latin translations:

- *Persea gratissima:* Avocado
- *Musa Sapientum:* Bananas (many different varieties have their own Latin name)
- *Bertholletia excelsa:* Brazil nut

- *Castanea sativa:* Chestnut (other varieties have their own Latin name)
- *Piscum iecur:* Fish liver oil
- *Actinidia chinensis:* Kiwi fruit (other varieties have their own Latin name)
- *Arachis hypogaea:* Peanut
- *Triticum vulgare:* Wheat

Medication

Certain medications can trigger anaphylaxis events in people with allergies, including the following:

- Allopurinol
- Anti-hypertensives
- Aspirin and non-steroidal anti-inflammatory drugs
- Blood products
- Insulin
- Muscle relaxants
- Radio-contrast media
- Penicillin and cephalosporin antibiotics
- Sulpha antibiotics
- Vaccines

Anaesthetists often ask patients, while they're being anaesthetised, whether they have a metallic taste in the mouth, because this taste is a tell-tale sign that a person's experiencing an allergic reaction to the anaesthetic.

Patients taking beta-blockers (a medication often used for heart disease or hypertension) can delay any mild allergic reactions to severe anaphylaxis (because the drug blocks part of the natural defence against anaphylaxis). When the serum levels of the drug wear off, however, the allergic reaction to the antigen springs into action.

Latex

Exposure to latex is commonly through the gloves used in healthcare. Many areas now use a latex-free variety of gloves, though latex gloves can still be found in operating theatres, because they're used during surgical operations. Therefore, patients who've had multiple operations/procedures are more likely to be sensitised to latex.

Other high-risk groups are individuals with dermatitis, asthma or those with food allergies. Patients allergic to certain fruits such as bananas and kiwi fruits, and vegetables such as avocados and potatoes, may also be allergic to latex, because these food items have similar protein chains to the rubber tree.

Here's the full list of fruit and vegetables with similar protein chains to latex:

- Apples
- Avocados
- Bananas
- Celery
- Cherries
- Chestnuts
- Ficus
- Figs
- Grapes
- Kiwi
- Mangoes
- Melons
- Passion Fruit
- Peaches
- Pears
- Pistachios
- Potatoes
- Ragweed
- Strawberries
- Tomatoes

Taking a Tour of the Bodily Systems Affected

Anaphylaxis (which I define in the earlier section 'Comparing allergies and anaphylaxis') can encroach on five bodily systems:

- Integumentary (cutaneous)
- Central nervous system
- Respiratory

 ✔ Gastrointestinal

 ✔ Cardiovascular

I cover each of these areas in turn in this section.

Impacting the integumentary system

Integumentary relates to the skin, hair and nails, but during an anaphylaxis event you can see the cutaneous reaction, which can result in the following:

 ✔ Itching (pruritis)

 ✔ Redness (erythema)

 ✔ Sweating

 ✔ Swelling to the airway and facial area (angio-oedema)

 ✔ Urticaria (hives)

Most patients who experience skin changes caused by an allergy don't go on to develop an anaphylactic reaction, but *they can do so.*

Angio-oedema is the swelling that occurs around the mouth, throat and face. The eyes may start to close due to this swelling. In the throat, *laryngeal oedema* occludes the airway to such an extent that the individual can no longer breathe. In the community, call an ambulance and explain that the person is having a severe allergic reaction. Paramedics on the scene may then have to facilitate tracheal intubation creating a mini tracheostomy (known as a *cricoidectomy*).

Striking at the central nervous system

Central nervous system reactions include the following:

 ✔ **Altered level of consciousness:** From the normal state of wakefulness and awareness to loss of consciousness.

 ✔ **Apprehension/Anxiety:** Possible early indicator of anaphylactic events.

 ✔ **Confusion:** Caused by decreased brain oxygenation and brain perfusion.

 ✔ **Faintness and dizziness:** Occurs due to hypotension.

✔ **Feeling of impending doom:** A strange phenomenon that indicates central nervous system involvement; patients have a feeling that they're going to die.

✔ **Metallic taste in mouth:** Often noted as an early symptom of anaphylactic events.

Loss of consciousness is a life-threatening symptom.

Affecting the respiratory system

Respiratory reactions can include the following:

✔ Dyspnoea (shortness of breath or breathlessness)

✔ Hypoxia (deficiency of oxygen to the tissues)

✔ Laryngeal obstruction leading to stridor

✔ Respiratory arrest

✔ Rhinitis (stuffy, blocked nose or a nose running profusely)

✔ Wheezing

Stridor is a high-pitched noise heard on inspiration and created by an upper airway obstruction. It may be caused by a head injury and is a medical emergency.

Hitting the gastrointestinal system

Gastrointestinal reactions can include the following:

✔ Abdominal cramps

✔ Diarrhoea

✔ Nausea

✔ Vomiting

The time of reaction affecting the gastrointestinal system depends on what the person was exposed to. For example, injections (especially IV injections) tend to have a quicker reaction than injected venom, which tends to have a quicker reaction than orally ingested triggers (for more on triggers, flip to the earlier 'Covering the causes of anaphylaxis' section).

Attacking the cardiovascular system

Cardiovascular reactions can include the following:

- Arrhythmias
- Cardiac arrest
- Hypotension
- Tachycardia

People's blood pressure falls and the pulse rate rises as they go into anaphylactic shock. Cardiovascular involvement is life-threatening and obtaining treatment quickly is vital. Symptoms present as for any signs of shock – a pale and clammy appearance and a feeling of faintness and dizziness.

Patients with anaphylaxis can deteriorate if made to sit up or stand up.

Managing Anaphylaxis Events

In the first instance, of course, managing anaphylaxis events is prevention: not exposing the individual to the antigen. Therefore, patients admitted to hospital need to have a thorough assessment, checking for any previous reactions to medications and so on, before prescribing and administering. After any new medication, or vaccination, individuals should be observed and remain in the location for 10 minutes (checking for any reaction).

If person does start to react, carry out these steps in the initial stages:

1. **Call for help and assess patient using the ABCDE approach – see Figure 13-1.**
2. **Lay the person flat.**
3. **Raise feet (you need to restore blood pressure).**
4. **Administer anaphylaxis drugs (such as adrenalin).**
5. **Reassure the person.**
6. **Document your actions.**

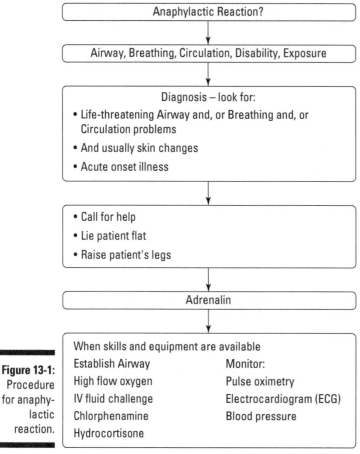

Figure 13-1: Procedure for anaphylactic reaction.

© John Wiley & Sons, Inc.

Knowing the right course of action

The flow chart in Figure 13-1 shows the course of action for when an individual is experiencing an anaphylactic reaction in a hospital environment.

Here's the ever-useful 'ABC' for detecting life-threatening problems:

- ✔ **Airway:** Swelling, hoarseness, stridor
- ✔ **Breathing:** Rapid breathing, wheeze, fatigue, cyanosis, SPO2 < 92%, confusion
- ✔ **Circulation:** Pale, clammy, low blood pressure, faintness, drowsy/coma

Here are the adrenalin doses (give intramuscularly [IM] unless experienced with adrenalin) – IM doses of 1:1,000 adrenalin (repeat after five minutes if no better):

- **Adult:** 500 micrograms IM (0.5 ml)
- **Child more than 12 years:** 500 micrograms IM (0.5 ml)
- **Child 6–12 years:** 300 micrograms IM (0.3ml)
- **Child less than 6 years:** 150 micrograms IM (0.15 ml)

Adrenalin IV is to be given only by experienced specialists – titrate: adults 50 micrograms; children 1 micrograms/kg.

The IV fluid challenge is administering IV fluids in order to replenish lost bodily fluid – sometimes referred to as *fluid resuscitation:*

- **Adult:** 500–1,000 ml; Hartman or Sodium Chloride 0.9%
- **Child:** Crystalloid 20 ml/kg

Stop IV colloid if it may be the cause of anaphylaxis.

Here are the doses if further drug therapy is deemed necessary:

Patient	Chlorphenamine (IM or slow IV)	Hydrocortisone (IM or slow IV)
Adult or child >12 years	10 mg	200 mg
Child 6–12 years	5 mg	100 mg
Child less than 6 years	2.5 mg	50 mg
Child less than 6 months	250 micrograms/kg	25 mg

Meeting adrenalin – the wonder drug

In the hospital environment, adrenalin (epinephrine) is known as the first line of emergency drugs in the treatment of anaphylaxis, and is presented as 1:1,000 ratio, which means that 1 millilitre of the volume has 1,000 micrograms of the drug (or 1 milligram).

The person experiencing the anaphylaxis requires 0.5 milligrams (500 micrograms = 0.5 millilitres) injection, followed by another 0.5 milligrams five minutes later if no clinical improvement. For children, this dose is reduced.

Under the Safer Patient Initiative, the adrenalin doesn't need to be prescribed, because the drug comes under a Patient Group Directive (PGD). The nurse administering the adrenalin needs to have signed this PGD document previously, be up-to-date on resuscitation training and be competent at delivering this treatment. Note, however, that practice does vary in different hospitals.

Administer adrenalin intramuscularly – usually to the mid-outer thigh area, due to its accessibility (the vastus lateralis muscle). You should also administer oxygen via a non-re-breather mask.

Hospitals tend to have an 'Anaphylaxis emergency box' containing the adrenalin. This box often also contains the following medication, known as the 'second line' of emergency drugs, which may need to be drawn up if not in a pre-filled syringe:

- 3 x 1ml adrenalin 1:1,000
- 1 x 10 ml aminophylline (250 mg in 10 ml) – to reverse airway obstruction
- 1 x 1 ml chlorphenamine (10 mg in 1 ml) – for the symptomatic relief of allergy, such as urticaria
- 1 x 100 mg hydrocortisone – for angio-oedema and anaphylactic shock
- 1 x 5 ml water for injection – to reconstitute the hydrocortisone, because this medication comes in a powder format

These *second line* drugs in the treatment for anaphylaxis need to be prescribed and don't come under the PGD.

In the community, adrenalin needs to be carefully stored, because it has to be protected from direct sunlight and extremes of temperature.

Some individuals carry an auto-injector (a pre-filled syringe). The adult dose is often smaller than a hospital dose, because these auto-injectors may contain 300 micrograms (0.3 milligrams) per injection rather than the 500 micrograms (0.5 milligrams). Children's doses tend to be smaller, in the region of 150 micrograms of adrenalin.

Seeing how adrenalin works

During the exposure to the troublesome antigen, a chemical cascade occurs within the body (such as histamines, cortisone and so on), which causes the swelling and runny eyes and so on. Anaphylaxis causes blood vessels to leak, bronchial tissues to swell and blood pressure to drop, causing choking and collapse.

Adrenalin (the wonder drug) acts quickly to:

- ✔ Constrict blood vessels
- ✔ Relax smooth muscles in the lungs to improve breathing
- ✔ Stimulate the heart's contractility
- ✔ Help to stop swelling around the face and lips (angio-oedema)

Considering after care

After everything has settled down and the patient is stable, give lots of reassurance and an information leaflet explaining anaphylaxis.

Even when the patient improves, continue to observe because the 'rebound' effect may kick in – technically known as the *biphasic response*. Rebound can occur even some hours later and the individual should be informed about this possibility and how to treat with further adrenalin if she's been sent home. You need to complete all the necessary documentation.

The GP or hospital doctor may request any of the following tests:

- ✔ **Blood tests:** These tests are a clotted blood sample: 5 ml of blood in adults (0.5 ml of blood in children) is collected in serum or clotted tubes and sent to immunology for mast cell tryptase 1–2 hours after the start of symptoms. Further samples should be collected and sent. Concentrations go back to normal within 6–8 hours.

  These samples don't tell patients what they're sensitive to, only that they had a reaction.

- ✔ **Urine tests:** The bladder should be emptied immediately after the reaction and then urine collected for 2–4 hours. This procedure is to measure methylhistamine, which is what histamine turns into when the body inactivates it.

- ✔ **Immunology therapy:** Small doses of the antigen are injected in the patient and they build up a resistance to the protein. These tests are conducted in highly controlled circumstances and the person is closely observed.

✔ **Skin prick tests:** To establish what the person was allergic to. Like blood tests, skin prick tests can show false negatives and false positives. These tests predict the likelihood of a specific food, or substance, causing a reaction, but they don't predict a reaction's severity.

✔ **Food challenges tests:** Where a person eats small amounts of the suspected allergen in a controlled environment. Gradually you increase the amounts until it's clear that she's not allergic: that is, when no reaction occurs. This challenge may also be conducted in the case of medication, whereby the prescribed drug is gradually increased over a period of time.

Reporting Adverse Reactions

Individuals experiencing allergic reactions to a trigger antigen should visit their GP as soon as possible after leaving hospital. They may be referred to an allergy clinic for further investigation. Sometimes the cause of the reaction isn't found, called *idiopathic anaphylaxis,* meaning 'cause unknown'.

Here I discuss what you need to do as a health professional to report an incident involving an adverse reaction.

Using the yellow card system

The yellow card scheme is a system in the UK for collecting suspected adverse drug reactions to medicines. The system is run by the Medicines and Healthcare Products Regulatory Agency (MHRA) and the Commission on Human Medicines (CHM). Doctors, nurses, patients, parents of children or carers can complete the yellow card – in short, anyone seeing or experiencing an adverse effect from any medication, however minor.

You can obtain the yellow cards from pharmacists, online, health centres and at the back of the British National Formulary, as a pull out/tear off.

Completing in-house documentation

If the allergic reaction is drug-related in a hospital environment, you need to complete all documentation according to policies and procedures of the individual healthcare environment. For example, for a reaction that occurs during a transfusion, you need to complete documentation relating to blood transfusion and resuscitation.

Reactions during transfusions

Although rare, anaphylactic reactions can occur during blood or plasma transfusions. They occur usually after the first few millilitres of the transfusion have been infused. Signs include the following:

- Abdominal cramps
- Bronchial spasm
- Respiratory distress
- Shock and potential loss of consciousness

The transfusion needs to be stopped immediately and resuscitation commence.

Part III
Figuring Out Infusion Rates for IV Therapy

Five ways to improve your skills when using infusion devices

- ✔ Practise working out infusion pump rates for when you're using syringe drivers and volumetric pumps.
- ✔ Master IV drip rates when using the gravity method of administration, so that it becomes second nature.
- ✔ Ensure that you're familiar with titrating drugs according to the patient's body weight.
- ✔ Rehearse infusing IV fluids safely through peripheral lines.
- ✔ Take onboard the great tips for infusing IV fluids efficiently through central lines.

Healthcare professionals infuse drugs regularly with IV therapy. Discover free articles about what you need to know about infusions at www.dummies.com/extras/nursingcalculationsandivtherapyuk.

In this part . . .

- ✔ Become aware of total body water amounts in order to maintain correct fluid balance in the body.

- ✔ Get to know the principles of infusing blood and blood components to ensure that you use these fluids safely.

- ✔ Understand the infection control principles to reduce infections when administering IV drugs, so that you maintain the patient's safety throughout the procedure.

- ✔ Be aware of the complications of IV therapy and adverse reactions in order to recognise when to intervene appropriately.

- ✔ Find out about the analgesic morphine, to ensure that you use it safely and correctly.

Chapter 14

Water, Water, Everywhere! Looking at IV Fluids

In This Chapter

▶ Staying on the right side of the law

▶ Watching fluids flow in the body

▶ Using IV drip equipment

*I*ntravenous (IV) therapy is the infusion of fluids such as 0.9% sodium chloride (administered to correct electrolyte unbalances and/or for hydration purposes) and liquid forms of medications such as IV amoxicillin (to treat infections), which go directly into the circulatory system – *intravenous* simply means 'within the vein'. These fluids come in many different forms from the manufacturer and are sterile to protect the recipient from pathogens.

The IV route is the fastest way to deliver fluids and medications throughout the body with a bioavailability of 100 per cent (as I discuss in Chapter 6). This rapid means of administration into the body's system, however, comes with complications. For instance, before you administer an IV fluid, you need to know whether you're using the correct fluid – infusing the wrong one can cause more harm than good in many cases. In other words, as I discuss in this chapter, what does the infusion need to do – target the inside, outside or around the cells in the body?

Fluids are administered for many different reasons, such as when a person has acute diarrhoea or vomiting and his fluid volume (known as *total body water*) falls. Heavy bleeding can also cause fluid volume depletion, requiring an IV blood transfusion. Electrolyte levels in the blood can also go haywire (technical term!) when fluid volume is decreased or increased, something that needs to be rectified with the correct replacement after clinical assessment.

Intravenous therapy can also be administered in order to deliver medications, such as antibiotics, chemotherapy drugs and/or parenteral nutrition. As with all drug administration, nurses require a factual knowledge of the drug: usual dosage, special considerations and common adverse effects. I look at all these aspects, plus the equipment used and the legal side of IV administration, in this chapter. For much more on IV therapy, check out Chapter 15.

Considering the Legal Aspects of IV

Patients who receive IV therapy have the right to expect safe care from appropriately trained and competent healthcare professionals. Therefore, you need to be deemed competent in mathematical ability, to have sufficient knowledge of the legal and professional issues (including your own personal accountability), and to maintain this competency over time.

Meeting the 'special ones' who can administer IV fluids

When administering IV drugs to patients, nurses, midwives, assistant practitioners, operating department practitioners, cardiac physiologists and so on are required to be competent in all clinical aspects of this skill.

Required expertise

In order to practise safely, you must have knowledge of the following:

- Legal and professional issues (including accountability)
- Pharmacology of giving drugs via the IV route (including contra-indications)
- Methods of administration and how to reconstitute drugs
- Drug calculations
- Total body water volume amounts and bodily fluid compartments (see the later sections 'Being aware of total body water volume' and 'Describing the fluid compartments', respectively)
- Fluid and electrolyte balance (see Chapter 15 for more on the latter)
- Blood transfusion procedures (see Chapter 17)
- Infection control
- Principles of IV access devices and care (see Chapter 16)

✔ Prevention and management of complications, including speed shock (Chapter 19), drug errors and anaphylaxis (Chapter 13)

✔ Correct documentation and good record keeping

The usual practice is for healthcare professionals to attend an intravenous study session after passing a drug calculations test. Doing so helps you to maintain your professional accountability and to be familiar with the documents: Nursing and Midwifery Council for Standards Medicines Management (2008) and the Royal College Nursing Standards for Infusion Therapy (2010). You also discover the local policies and procedures of your employer relating to IVs and medication administration.

Professional accountability also requires you to check and be certain of the following:

✔ The identity of the patient receiving the medication

✔ That the patient isn't allergic to the medicine before you administer it

✔ The therapeutic uses of the medicine to be administered – its normal dosage, side effects, precautions and contra-indications

✔ The patient's care plan and medical notes

✔ What the prescription chart is asking for (for example, method of administration, route and timing)

✔ That the medicine label is clearly readable

✔ That the medication expiry date hasn't passed

✔ That the correct calculations for dosage and weight (where appropriate) have been obtained and checked

✔ Whether you should withhold medication due to the patient's condition (for example, digoxin can't be administered if the pulse rate is below 60 beats per minute)

✔ Actions to be taken if contra-indications to a medication are observed, as well as the correct actions for drug errors

✔ Signing all relevant documentation where medicine has been administered, intentionally withheld or refused by patient

Relevant formula

Sometimes you need to add (by injecting) a drug into a bag of IV fluids, such as in the case of severe infection: for example, 1 gram of IV Amoxicillin into a 500-millilitre IV bag of sodium chloride 0.9% to be infused over 60 minutes. The IV infusion bag needs to have a label on it indicating the bag of sodium chloride 0.9% also has 1 gram of amoxicillin added within this bag.

The formula for working out the liquid dosage to administer is the same one that you use for administering bolus IV injections and for oral ingestion of drugs – in short, you use this formula for working out liquid amounts, whatever the route of administration:

$$\text{What you want} \Big/ \text{What you've got} \times \text{Volume}$$

A patient is prescribed naloxone 0.6 mg IV. Stock ampoules contain 0.4 mg/2 ml. What volume do you need to draw up?

Use the formula in the preceding paragraph:

$$0.6/0.4 \times 2 \text{ ml} = 3 \text{ ml}$$

Chapter 16 looks at the means of getting fluids into the bloodstream (the IV system access devices) and Chapter 8 describes the calculations that you need to master in order to administer liquid dosages of medication for injections.

Watching for adverse drug reactions

Drugs, such as IV antibiotics, are very often added to the IV bags of fluids to be administered by continuous infusion. The healthcare professional needs knowledge and understanding of the IV drug as well as the intravenous fluid. The first step in the safe administration of any IV drug, as in all drug administration, is to become familiar with the drug, the patient's medical history and being aware of the potential for *adverse drug reactions* (ADRs). Note that not many drugs are given by IV bolus (one-off IV injection) as the preferred method.

Adverse drug reactions are unexpected side effects of taking medication that tend not to be predicted, unlike allergic reactions involving the immune system (see Chapter 13). For example, if a patient feels sick after taking a new medication, the cause is more likely to be an adverse reaction to the drug. If the same patient experiences shortness of breath and angio-oedema, an allergic reaction to the drug is more likely.

Many of your patients, the over-65s in particular, may take four or more medications per day. Known as *polypharmacy,* this can give rise to increased incidents of ADR, due to the potential for creating a toxic drug combination.

You need to assess predisposing factors that could increase the risk of ADR prior to administering any medication to the patient, in order to ensure the person's safety: for example, patient's age, gender, ethnic origin, genetic factors, allergies and intolerances, and state of health.

Drug-to-drug interactions are another potential for causing ADR, because many medications shouldn't be prescribed together, such as the following:

- ✔ **Erythromycin (for infections in patients with penicillin hypersensitivity) and amlodipine (for hypertension):** A possible side effect can increase low blood pressure effects.

- ✔ **Warfarin (for treating venous thrombosis) and amiodarone hydrochloride (cardiac arrhythmias):** A possible side effect can increase anticoagulant effects.

- ✔ **Morphine (an opioid analgesic – see Chapter 20) and imipramine hydrochloride (for depressive illness and nocturnal enuresis (night-time bed wetting in children):** A possible side effect can increase sedation and narcotic effects.

- ✔ **Fentanyl (for severe chronic pain) and promethazine hydrochloride (for symptomatic relief of allergy):** A possible side effect can increase central nervous system and respiratory depressive effects.

Crossover reactions can also cause ADR. This situation arises because patients with a known allergy to a particular drug can be at risk of having an allergic reaction to a different drug with a similar chemical structure: for example, the anti-epileptic medication phenytoin with other drugs of the central nervous system, such as barbiturates.

Staying within the law: Vicarious liability

Vicarious liability is a legal term, which in short states how you need to work within the law and your job contract. Your employer takes liability for any actions and omissions, as long as you act within the job description and boundaries that the employer has approved.

As a nurse, I know that I can only administer IV medications after I've been on a study session for IV therapy and anaphylaxis, passed my IV drug calculations test and been deemed competent of performing this skill. Without this knowledge base and skills in place, I'd be breaking vicarious liability. In other words, I can't legally perform this clinical skill.

Understanding Fluids in the Body

In this section I look at IV fluid replacement, which includes needing to know a little about total body water amounts and the fluid compartments.

I describe fluid balance in Chapter 7 – how the body strives to maintain homeostasis by matching the fluid intake to the fluid output. An alteration in one of these disrupts this equilibrium, leading to fluid and electrolyte imbalance (see Chapter 15).

Being aware of total body water volume

The *total body water amount* (TBW) is the percentage of lean body weight. It varies with age and the amount of fat, because the latter has a much lower water content than muscle. As a result, TBW as a percentage of total body weight is lower in individuals with more fat.

Here are the approximate normal values of TBW:

- **Premature infants:** 80%
- **Term infants:** 70–75%
- **Toddlers:** 65–70%
- **After puberty and adulthood:** 60%

Staying hydrated

To maintain balance, the body acquires fluids and electrolytes through the intake of food and drink and loses fluids and electrolytes through four bodily organs:

- **Kidneys:** Maintain urine output of approximately 1–2 litres per day in a healthy adult, though less may be produced during illness.
- **Skin:** A healthy adult loses between 350–450 millilitres of fluid daily through the skin. Fever increases sweating and burns can increase the loss.
- **Lungs:** An adult can lose 300–400 millilitres of water vapour through the lungs per day. Patients with *tachypnoea* (a fast breathing rate) lose more and patients on ventilators much less.
- **Gastrointestinal tract (GI):** The intestines reabsorb most of the fluid taken into the body, and so only 100–200 millilitres of fluid are lost through the GI tract. During episodes of diarrhoea, this loss increases.

Having too much or too little fluid

Clinical consequences result if a patient has too much fluid – *hypervolaemia* – or too little – *hypovolaemia*.

Hypervolaemia is where the body experiences fluid overload, within the circulatory system, which produces an increase in the extracellular fluid volume (referred to as a *positive balance*). It can occur due to mismanagement of prescribed fluids and may cause pulmonary oedema and cardiac failure.

Signs to alert you of hypervolaemia in your patient include the following:

- ✔ Abnormal accumulation of fluid in the abdomen – known as *ascites*
- ✔ Decrease in blood urea nitrogen (BUN) measurements
- ✔ Decrease in serum sodium and osmolarity measurements
- ✔ Increase in the urine's specific gravity
- ✔ Increased need for urination – known as polyuria
- ✔ Oedema
- ✔ Weight gain

Hypovolaemia is when the bodily fluid loss exceeds the fluid intake over a period of time due to a decrease in extracellular fluid volume (referred to as a *negative balance*). It's commonly caused by dehydration and excessive fluid loss through bleeding or overuse of diuretics. Other causes include surgery, prolonged bouts of diarrhoea and vomiting, or severe burns.

The following signs alert you to possible hypovolaemia in your patient:

- ✔ Acute weight loss
- ✔ Altered mental status
- ✔ Clammy skin
- ✔ Dark, concentrated urine
- ✔ Decreased central venous pressure
- ✔ Decreased skin *turgor* (ability of the skin to return to its normal shape when gently pinched)
- ✔ Decreased urine output *(oliguria)*
- ✔ Flattened jugular veins when lying down
- ✔ Hypotension in usually normotensive patients
- ✔ Thirst
- ✔ Weak rapid pulse

Flip to the later section 'Treating hypovolaemic shock' for dealing with serious cases.

Monitoring your patient

Assessing and monitoring fluid balance is a key element of patient care. It comprises keeping vigilant fluid balance input and output records and assessing the following items:

- ✔ Arterial blood gas results
- ✔ Capillary refill
- ✔ Central venous pressure (CVP) measurements
- ✔ Daily weight
- ✔ Jugular vein filling
- ✔ Serum electrolyte levels
- ✔ Skin turgor
- ✔ Urine specific gravity
- ✔ Vital signs – respirations, pulse, blood pressure, temperature and recording them on the National Early Warning Score (NEWS) chart

You can use the skin turgor test to assess for dehydration. Gently pinch skin from the back of the patient's hand between two fingers so that it's tented up and held for a few seconds before being released. Skin with normal skin turgor snaps back rapidly, whereas skin with decreased skin turgor remains elevated and only slowly returns to its normal position.

Check out Chapter 19 for more on hypervolaemia caused by IV infusion.

Describing the fluid compartments

The total body water has two main compartments, which are separated by a cell membrane, through which the body water can easily pass:

- ✔ **Extracellular fluid**: Outside the body cell
- ✔ **Intracellular fluid:** Inside the body cell

The sizes of these two main compartments vary with age, with the extracellular compartment being increased in infants and young children, compared to older people. The cell membrane separating the compartments is freely permeable to water, but not to electrolytes and other large molecules.

Intracellular space is the space within all body cells and *extracellular space* is the space outside of the cells. The extracellular compartment can be further divided into *intravascular space,* which is the space within the blood vessels, and the *interstitial space,* which is the space between the cells (but not within the blood vessels).

The breakdown of the body's fluid, within the body, is known as the *60-40-20* rule: 60 per cent of the human body weight is water, 40 per cent of this is intracellular fluids and 20 per cent of this is made up of extracellular fluid (60 per cent in total).

Transporting the fluids

If you're wondering how the water moves into or outside the cells, you must be psychic, because that's what I discuss now! Like with any long journey, you need transport.

Movement of water within the body follows four key principles of molecule transport modes:

- ✔ **Osmosis:** Body water is generally pulled towards a solution with a higher concentration of dissolved molecules. Osmosis is the movement of water across a semi-permeable membrane that selectively allows certain structures to pass while inhibiting others. The osmotic movement of water occurs as the body attempts to create a balance that exists on either side of the membrane. The water easily crosses the semi-permeable membrane from the side that has a lower concentration of particles to the side with a higher concentration of particles. This movement stops when each side of the membrane becomes equal in its concentration of water and particles.

- ✔ **Diffusion:** Where a movement of solutes (a substance) move across the semi-permeable membrane from an area of high concentration to an area of low concentration. Diffusion is a passive transport mechanism, meaning that it doesn't require any energy. When the diffused particles are evenly distributed, resulting in an equal concentration on either side of the membrane, the movement stops.

- ✔ **Active transport:** Sometimes a cell needs a higher concentration of one ion on one side of the membrane than on the other, as in the case of sodium and potassium. The movement of a substance across a membrane from a region of lower concentration to a region of higher concentration against a gradient using energy is known as active transport. In other words, the transport requires energy synthesised within the cell, as in the case of the sodium/potassium pump.

- ✔ **Facilitated diffusion:** The movement of solutes from an area of high concentration to an area of low concentration, facilitated by a carrier molecule. An example is glucose entering the cell in the presence of insulin.

Therefore, before you start administering IV fluids, you need to understand the patient's fluid replacement requirements and how these fluids work to preserve equilibrium.

Knowing the types of IV fluids

Intravenous fluids include the *volume expanders* (IV infusions that provide volume to the circulatory system) and include crystalloids and colloids (*isotonic* effective volume expanders for short periods of time and so good for hypotensive and hypovolaemic patients), blood-based products, blood substitutes, medication (including buffer solutions used to correct acidosis or alkalosis within the body) and nutrition:

- **Crystalloid:** Aqueous solutions of mineral salts or other water-soluble molecules that contain electrolytes (see Chapter 15). Crystalloids tend to create low osmotic pressure, allowing fluids to move across the blood vessels, which can therefore be linked to oedema. They tend to be much cheaper than colloids (blood, albumin, plasma and so on). Crystalloids are categorised into three types according to their osmolarity compared with plasma osmolarity:

  - *Isotonic solutions:* Have the same osmolarity to plasma. An example is 0.9% sodium chloride. They can be helpful in treating hypotensive or hypovolaemic patients.

    Isotonic solutions are where fluids stay where they're put.

  - *Hypotonic solutions:* Have a lower osmolarity than plasma. An example is 0.45% sodium chloride. Ringer's lactate is a mildly hypotonic solution often used in patients with severe burns. These solutions can be helpful for hyperglycaemic conditions, such as diabetic keto-acidosis where high serum levels draw fluid out of the cells.

    Hypotonic solutions are where fluids move out of the vessel (the fluid quickly moves from the blood vessels into the cells).

  - *Hypertonic solutions:* Have a higher osmolarity than plasma. An example is 5% dextrose. They can be used post-operatively to help stabilise blood pressure, increase urine output and reduce oedema.

    Hypertonic solutions enter the vessel (the fluid pulls water from the cells into the blood vessels).

- **Colloid:** These products contain larger particles (usually proteins) that aren't soluble in water such as gelatin and albumin (plasma protein), and therefore create high osmotic pressure, attracting fluids into the blood vessels. Colloid molecules are large and last longer in the intravascular fluid compartment than crystalloids, and so less fluid volume may be required. This fact can help in reducing oedema (such as pulmonary or cerebral oedema) while expanding the intravascular volume. Colloids are derived from natural sources within the body, such as albumin and synthetic solutions: for example, gelatins.

✔ **Blood-based products:** Blood products are hypertonic and an example of a commonly administered intravenous colloid in cases of massive blood loss due to trauma or surgery. People with sickle-cell disease may require frequent blood transfusions. Blood can also be used to treat severe cases of anaemia or thrombocytopenia.

Thrombocytopenia indicates an abnormally low number of platelets in the blood (platelets are called *thromobocytes*). Normal platelet count is approximately 150,000 to 450,000 platelets per microlitre of blood: a count below 150,000 is therefore lower than normal (called *thrombocytopenia*). Chemotherapy drugs often lower the platelet count of individuals.

✔ **Blood substitutes:** Artificial substances that aim to provide an alternative to blood-based products acquired from donors.

✔ **Buffer solutions:** These solutions rectify acid-base imbalance – that is, they correct acidosis or alkalosis. Lactated ringer's solution also has some buffering effect, but the main buffering solution is intravenous sodium bicarbonate.

✔ **Medications:** Certain medications can only be administered via the IV route, such as intravenous immunoglobulin and propofol. Some medications may also require mixing with other fluids to dilute their concentration, such as 0.9% sodium chloride plus 5% dextrose. Some IV medications are mixed in a syringe with water for injection or sodium chloride 0.9%, such as insulin or heparin to be administered IV via a syringe driver pump: more about these medications in Chapter 15.

IV fluids such as 0.9% sodium chloride comprise solutes dissolved in a solvent.

✔ **Parenteral nutrition:** Intravenous nutrition, which bypasses the usual process of eating and digestion. The IV nutrition formula contain proteins, carbohydrates, lipids, vitamins, minerals and trace elements as well as electrolytes. This IV solution can be customised to match the patient's requirements. *Total Parenteral Nutrition* (TPN) is where the patient receives all his nutrition via this means, whereas *Peripheral Parenteral Nutrition* (PPN) is where the patient receives only a portion of daily nutrition through a peripheral line IV.

Many of the nutrition preparations are light-sensitive and so you need to cover them during administration.

✔ **Chemotherapy:** A specialised form of IV drug administration requiring extended training, although chemotherapy can also be administered via different routes, such as orally or intrathecally. Intravenous chemotherapy can also be administered via a direct bolus into a tumour, organ or extremity. Chemotherapy drugs, called *cytotoxins,* kill off the rapidly dividing malignant cells, but also unfortunately the rapidly dividing normal cells, such as gastrointestinal cells and hair follicles (hence the often unpleasant side effects of nausea and vomiting and hair loss). Many chemotherapy drugs are added to IV infusions for slow continuous administration.

Table 14-1 lists some of the more commonly used IV fluids.

Table 14-1	Common IV Fluids
Type of IV Fluid	*Clinical Use*
0.9% sodium chloride	Suitable for resuscitation in hypovolaemic shock. Fluid of choice for routine maintenance and patients with head injury.
4.5% human albumin solution	Alternative for 0.9% sodium chloride for resuscitation in hypovolaemic shock.
0.9% sodium chloride + 5% dextrose	Suitable for maintenance fluid therapy in infants and children requiring isotonic fluid and for patients with hypoglycaemia. Can also be given peripherally to expand volume in varying situations.
0.45% sodium chloride + 5% dextrose	Suitable for maintenance fluid therapy in infants and children.
0.45% sodium chloride + 10% dextrose	Suitable for maintenance fluid therapy in infants and children with hypoglycaemia.
Hartmann's solution	Suitable for children undergoing surgery – for intra-operative and post-operative use.
0.18% sodium chloride + 4% dextrose	Not recommended for routine maintenance.
10% dextrose in water	A concentrated formula that can be given peripherally to treat hypoglycaemia.
3% sodium chloride	Used primarily in emergency situations, such as treating hyponatraemia (especially when seizures present). Must be administered slowly and with caution.

Routine maintenance of IV fluid and electrolyte replacement consists of giving the following three dosages:

✔ 25–30 ml/kg/day of water

✔ Approximately 1 mmol/kg/day of potassium, sodium and chloride

✔ Approximately 50–100 g/day of glucose to limit starvation ketosis

Treating hypovolaemic shock

Losing approximately one fifth or more of your total body water volume causes *hypovolaemic shock,* which results in the circulatory system becoming too depleted to perfuse adequately the tissues of the body. The aim of resuscitation in this instance is to correct the hypovolaemia and hypo-perfusion of the vital organs before irreversible damage occurs.

Testing whether fluid resuscitation is needed

Two tests to assess for hypovolaemic shock and decreased peripheral perfusion are the capillary refill time (CRT) and passive leg-raising tests:

✔ **Capillary refill time:** This test is conducted by raising the patient's hand higher than heart level and pressing on it to exert external pressure for a few seconds until the area turns white. After pressure is released, capillary refill time is the time it takes for the colour to return to the area. Normal capillary refill time is 2 seconds for adults and children and approximately 3 seconds for newborns. A prolonged capillary refill time

is usually a sign of shock and can indicate dehydration and decreased peripheral perfusion.

✔ **Passive leg-raising test:** This test is conducted to evaluate the need for fluid resuscitation in critically ill patients. It involves the patient raising his legs, which causes gravity to pull blood from the legs to increase circulatory volume, with the maximum effect occurring between 30–90 seconds. You then assess blood pressure and heart rates to make a clinical judgement as to whether more fluids need to be prescribed and administered.

To assess for serious hypovolaemia and the need for urgent fluid resuscitation, the initial assessment consists of information gathering for the following urgent indicators:

✔ Systolic blood pressure is less than 100 mmHg

✔ Heart rate is more than 90 beats per minute

✔ Capillary refill time is more than 2 seconds or peripheries are cold to the touch

✔ Respiratory rate is more than 20 breaths per minute

✔ National Early Warning Score (NEWS) is 5 or more

✔ Passive leg-raising test is positive

The sidebar 'Testing whether fluid resuscitation is needed' describes the capillary refill time and passive leg-raising tests.

Management of fluid resuscitation consists of the following actions:

1. **Give high-flow oxygen, obtain IV access (large bore), identify the cause of the deficit and respond to it.**

2. **Administer a fluid bolus of 500 ml crystalloid solution.**

3. **Reassess the patient using the ABCDE approach (Airway, Breathing, Circulation, Disability, Exposure).**

4. **Check that the patient has received 2,000 ml of fluid replacement, if assessed as requiring further fluid resuscitation (if fluid replacement is less than 2,000 ml, administer a further fluid bolus of 250–500 ml of crystalloid solution).**

Tooling up for IV Drips

Administering IV fluids safely obviously involves having a complete understanding of the equipment and methods used. This section provides your one-stop-shop for this info. The precise piece of equipment and the method required often depends on whether the fluid is a 'clear fluid', such as sodium chloride, or a 'thickened fluid', such as packed red blood cells. These administration sets are different: the former delivers 20 drops per millilitre and the latter, which contains a filter, delivers 15 drops per millilitre.

You never administer blood and IV fluids containing potassium via the gravity method (in other words, without a pump): always go through a pump for safety.

Setting up IV administration sets for clear fluids

In this section, I give you a rundown on all the parts of the IV administration set. (I show how to work out the drip rate for clear fluids in the later 'Calculating drip rates using the gravity method' section.)

Check out Figure 14-1, which shows a 1-litre bag of sodium chloride being administered using the gravity method of administration. The IV fluid is simply hung on to a drip stand and delivered without an electronic pump. The nurse can adjust the flow rate using a roller clamp, to run faster or slower.

Most IV bags of fluid come premixed in bags from anything from 50 to 1,000 millilitres (1 litre). The IV tubing has several important parts to it. Figure 14-2 shows a fluid administration set.

Drip chamber

The drip chamber is just below the spike used to pierce the bag. This chamber is where you can count the number of drops dripping down from the bag over a period of one minute to obtain the all-important *drip rate*. The drip-rate calculation depends on the size of the bag of fluid and the type of fluid.

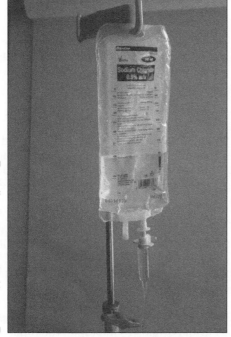

Figure 14-1:
A bag of
clear fluids
being
adminis-
tered via the
gravity
method (that
is, without a
pump).

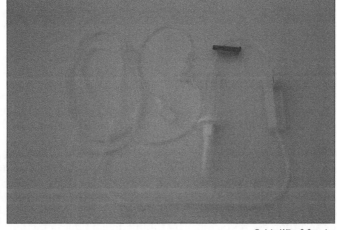

Figure 14-2:
Fluid admin-
istration set.

Count the number of drops over just 15 seconds and then multiply that number by four to get the number of drops in a full minute.

The drip chamber must always be half full, because if the chamber is too full you can't see the drops to count them. If the drip chamber isn't full enough, air can get into the tubing and in turn enter the patient's circulatory system, blocking a blood vessel and potentially stopping the heart.

Roller clamp

The roller clamp is where you control the rate at which the IV fluid infuses. Rolling it one way squeezes the tubing, making the fluid flow through the tubing more slowly. Rolling the roller clamp in the opposite direction loosens the pinching effect, making the tubing less narrow and allowing the fluid to run through the tubing faster.

If you work out that the drip rate is to be 15 drops per minute (dpm), from an initial rate of 22 dpm, you need to slow the rate down using the roller clamp.

If you want the drip rate to be 25 dpm from an initial rate of 14 dpm, you speed the rate up using the clamp.

When you initially set up the IV administration set, the roller clamp should be closed before attaching the bag of IV fluids to the top of the tubing, to ensure that no air gets into the tubing. You then need to *prime the line:* that is, fill it with fluid from the prescribed bag.

Doctors prescribe IV fluids over a set period of time and so nurses then need to work out the specific rate to deliver the fluids in the correct timeframe – known as the *infusion rate* or *flow rate*.

Slide clamp

The slide clamp is used to stop the infusion from flowing completely, without using the roller clamp. To use the slide clamp, you pinch the tubing completely shut when you slide the tubing into the narrowest part of the clamp.

The slide clamp comes into its own when you just need to turn the infusion off for a very short while and don't want to reset the flow rate using the roller clamp. When the slide clamp is pushed off from the tubing, the calculated flow rate continues as before. This is useful when the patient needs to get dressed and the infusion bag and tubing have to go through the sleeve of a jumper and then get restarted. The tubing doesn't get detached from the cannula with the potential of introducing bugs.

Injection port

The injection port along the line of the administration set is where you can add medicines or fluids, if they've not been added to the port on the fluid bag already.

The injection port on the bag of fluid mixes the fluid and drug, whereas the injection port on the IV line gives the patient drugs in a much more concentrated form because this port is *not* mixed.

Putting together IV administration sets for blood and thickened fluids

Setting up a bag of blood or blood products to administer is technically similar to setting up clear fluids drug administration (see the preceding section), except that these administration sets have a filter with two chambers and deliver 15 drops per millilitre rather than 20 drops per millilitre. (Make your way to Chapter 16 for all about the different IV access devices and Chapter 17 to see the special protocols that apply to the administration of blood and blood products.)

Whether you're administering a clear fluid, such as sodium chloride 0.9%, or a bag of packed red blood cells, you need to prime the administration set line, after you've checked that the patient's access device is *patent* (the line is open and not blocked) and good to go.

Never use dextrose/glucose preparations before or after blood administration, because it causes clumping of the cells. Best practice is to have a dedicated line for blood transfusions only. Where intravenous dextrose has been administered, you need to flush the cannula with sodium chloride prior to a blood transfusion.

To prime the line, if using a Baxter IV blood administration set, follow these steps:

1. **Use the roller to close the line.**
2. **Hold the bag inverted and spike the port.**
3. **Use the roller to open the line while keeping the bag inverted.**
4. **Squeeze the bag gently to fill the filter chamber completely.**
5. **Continue until the second chamber is half full.**
6. **Close the line using the roller.**
7. **Turn the bag and set the right way up.**
8. **Continue to prime the set to the end of the line by opening the roller.**

This method reduces frothing of the blood during priming and by completely covering the filter excludes air, which can promote clot formation.

Using a burette

You use a *volume-controlled burette* to administer relatively small amounts of volumes for dilution. This device is often used when dealing with infants and small children, whose fluid volume requirements are much smaller than adults. You can also use the device for fluid-restricted renal patients, where fluid volumes also need to be very precise – the rationale for always administering the fluids/medications through a pump.

These devices have a roller clamp at the top of the burette so that a bag of IV fluid can be attached above the burette. The burette has calibrated markings (for example, 1 millilitre apart) on the side. You can add the medication via an injection port at the top of the device and mix it with any dilutant required, from the bag attached above the burette device.

You can fill the burette with the correct fluid amount and then open it again to allow more fluid through if you need to mix a second dose of medication with the IV fluid.

Becoming proficient in using pump administration devices

Electronic infusion pumps use positive pressure to deliver IV fluids. The two types of electronic infusion pumps are *volumetric pumps* (also known as infusion pumps) and *syringe drivers* (also known as *syringe pumps*).

Electronic pumps enable you to deliver the fluid at a set and constant rate. Models vary from area to area, however, and so constant training is required when new devices are purchased.

Volumetric pumps generally involve you entering the volume and the prescribed timing for the infusion to be infused and the device sets the rate in millilitres/hour. You need to check these devices regularly: even when the cannula has been dislodged, the fluid continues to be delivered to the patient but into the surrounding tissue instead of the vein, known as *infiltration* (see Chapter 19).

For syringe drivers, the plunger of the syringe is controlled within the device – that is, controlling at what rate the syringe is being depressed and thereby at what rate and time the patient receives this medication. In the case of insulin, you can then adjust the rate according to the patient's condition, known as *a sliding scale:* for example, increasing the rate from 2 millilitres an hour to 2.5 millilitres hour, or decreasing the rate as required.

If you're asked to work out the rate to set the syringe driver, use the following formula to get an answer in millilitres per hour:

Volume (ml)/Time

A patient is to receive 24 millilitres of medication over 12 hours. The rate required for setting the syringe driver is as follows:

24 ml/12 hours = 2 ml/hour

The patient-controlled analgesia (PCA) device is another type of pump, which gives the patient control over his analgesic medication, simply by pressing a button and receiving a dose. These systems have a 'lock out' system, which means that patients shouldn't overdose, ensuring that they receive a set amount of the IV drug only at set time intervals and giving a total amount of the drug in a one- to four-hour timeframe.

If a patient requests the medication more frequently than allowed, the machine doesn't dispense the dose, but the information regarding the number of times the patient requests the analgesia can be recorded. From this information, the patient's pain relief medication can be adjusted.

Calculating drip rates using the gravity method

When the IV infusion is set up and the administration line primed, you can administer the IV fluids.

Drip rates

If you're delivering the fluids using the gravity method, here's the formula for working out the drip rate of clear fluids such as 0.9 % sodium chloride:

Drops per minute = Volume (ml)/Time (in hours) × Drops per ml/Minutes per hour (60)

Blood and clear fluids use different administration sets (often referred to as 'giving sets'):

- ✔ **Blood and thickened fluids use filtered giving sets:** 15 drops/ml
- ✔ **Clear fluids use standard giving sets:** 20 drops/ml
- ✔ **Microdrip or paediatric giving sets (sometimes referred to as a microdrop burette):** 60 drops/ml

Your patient has been prescribed 1 litre of 5% glucose to run over eight hours. Here's how to work out the drip rate in minutes per hour, using a standard administration set:

$$\frac{1{,}000 \text{ ml}}{8 \text{ hours}} \times 20 / 60 = 41.6 = 42 \text{ drops per minute to the nearest drop}$$

You need to give 420 millilitres of blood to a patient over four hours using a blood administration set. You work out the drip rate as follows:

$$\frac{420 \text{ ml}}{4 \text{ hours}} \times 15 / 60 = 26.25 = 26 \text{ drops per minute to the nearest drop}$$

Infusion process

Here are the steps for giving an IV fluid infusion:

1. **Collect all equipment.**

2. *Wash your hands.*

3. **Wear gloves (sterile gloves aren't required) if giving antibiotic therapy. Best practice calls for two nurses to check IV calculations.**

4. **Apply aseptic-non-touch-technique principles (ANTT; see Chapter 1) throughout the procedure.**

5. **Check that you have the correct patient and gain consent.**

6. **Inspect the fluid bag to be certain that it contains the correct fluid, the fluid is clear (if the medication should be), the bag isn't leaking and the date on the bag isn't expired.**

7. **Check that sterile packaging isn't damaged or wet.**

8. **Ensure that you have the correct giving set for the fluid to be administered (different sets are required for blood and blood products and electronic devices).**

   These sets are *microdrip* sets – which deliver 60 drops per ml into the drip chamber, or *macrodrip* sets – which deliver 15 to 20 drops per ml into the drip chamber.

9. **Open packaging and uncoil the tubing – don't let the ends of the tubing become contaminated.**

10. **Close the flow regulator (roll the wheel away from the end you'll attach to the fluid bag).**

11. **Remove the protective covering from the port of the fluid bag and the protective covering from the spike of the administration set.**

12. **Insert the spike of the administration set into the port of the fluid bag with a quick twist.**

Do Step 12 carefully. Be especially careful not to puncture yourself! Insert this spike fully into the infusion bag, because doing this task is an infection risk.

13. **Hold the fluid bag higher than the drip chamber of the administration set.**

14. **Squeeze the drip chamber once or twice to start the flow, filling the drip chamber to one-third full.**

If you overfill the chamber, lower the bag below the level of the drip chamber and squeeze some fluid back into the fluid bag.

15. **Open the flow regulator and allow the fluid to flush all the air from the tubing, letting it run into the giving set empty packaging or container.**

You may need to loosen or remove the cap at the end of the tubing to get the fluid to flow to the end of the tubing (though doing so shouldn't be necessary). Take care not to let the tip of the administration set become contaminated.

The primed giving set is now ready to be connected to an electronic device, or you can determine the rate by gravity flow together with the flow clamp.

16. **Connect the end of the tubing to the patient.**

The IV cannula must be of an appropriate size for the intended use and to minimise infection risk cleaned with a swab containing alcohol and chlorhexidine, and allowed to dry, before the giving set end is attached.

Working out the duration of a bag of IV fluids

When administering IV bags of fluids using the gravity method, you may sometimes need to work out how long the bag of fluid has left to run. The formula is similar to the formula for working out the drip rate in minutes per hour from the preceding section:

$$\text{Drip rate duration} = \frac{\text{Volume left in bag (ml)}}{\text{Rate of Infusion}} \times \text{Drops per ml} / 60 \text{ minutes}$$
$$(\text{drops per minute})$$

A patient has 600 millilitres of thickened fluids (fluid left in his IV bag to be infused, having already had 400 millilitres from the 1-litre bag prescribed). The IV drip rate was set at 20 drops per minute. You work out the time left for the infusion as follows:

$$\frac{600 \text{ ml}}{20 \text{ dpm}} = 15 \text{ drops per ml} / 60 \text{ minutes} = 7.5 = 7\frac{1}{2} \text{ hours}$$

Sometimes you may have to adjust the drip rate when administering IV fluids, slowing it down or speeding it up.

A patient is to have 3 litres of clear fluid over a time span of 24 hours. He has received 1,500 millilitres in 8 hours. How many drops per minute are required to correct the infusion?

Fluid left to infuse = 3,000 ml – 1,500 ml = 1,500 ml

Time left to infuse = 24 hours – 8 hours = 16 hours

$$\text{Drops per minute} = \frac{\text{Volume (ml)}}{\text{Time (in hours)}} \times \text{Drops per ml} / \text{Minutes per hour (60)}$$

$$\frac{1,500 \text{ ml}}{16 \text{ hours}} \times 20 \text{ dpm} / 60 = 31.25 = 31 \text{ drops per minute}$$

Chapter 15

Discussing Drips and Drops: IV Therapy

In This Chapter

▶ Knowing your IV therapy

▶ Administrating from ampoules and vials

▶ Considering continuous infusions – insulin and heparin

*I*ntravenous (IV) medicines and infusions are both types of IV drugs that enter the circulatory system through a peripheral or central vein.

IV infusions (solutions) may be given to rectify imbalances of electrolytes (salts and minerals in the body). Sometimes a drug may need to be reconstituted from a powder format to enable it to be administered through the IV route. The drug can then be added to a bag of IV fluid or given as injection – known as an IV bolus.

Some IV medicines need to be administered over a set time span as a continuous infusion, such as insulin and heparin, through a device known as a syringe driver.

I talk you through all these aspects of IV therapy in this chapter.

Looking at Methods of IV Therapy

Many different types of IV medications exist, as do methods of administering these drugs. I explore these methods in this section.

Considering IV drug methods

You need to understand the terms used for the various different ways of administering drugs via IV. Here are the three main methods and the different types of IV medication:

- **Bolus:** A single injection of a substance. This method of administration is sometimes referred to as a 'bolus push' or direct intermittent injection. Small volumes of the drug (usually up to a maximum of 20 millilitres) are directly administered into the peripheral or central venous access device or also via the injection port on an IV administration bag to be mixed with the solution.

  You have to give many of these drugs over a set period of time, unless in emergency situations, such as three to ten minutes, depending on the drug. Bolus injections cause an immediate 'peak' blood serum concentration, and so they're more likely to cause a reaction. Examples of medications that may be administered by bolus injection include IV furosemide and IV amoxicillin.

- **Continuous infusions:** Highly diluted medications, administered at a constant rate over a prescribed period of time, in order to deliver a controlled therapeutic response. The prescribed time can be anything from a couple of hours to several days.

  An example of a medication administered by continuous infusion is 1 litre of sodium chloride 0.9% given over eight hours. A bolus injection of another drug can be added to the 1-litre bag of sodium chloride and so on, but the bag must be labelled and mixed well to prevent a layering effect – that is, receiving the drug additive in one hit rather than mixed into the dilution (see Chapter 19 for details). Remember that bags of fluid are IV infusions, but they're also IV drugs – just in bigger volume.

  Heparin is a medication that you can administer by continuous infusion via a syringe driver pump. Two continuous infusions can be administered simultaneously using a Y connector, such as insulin (via a syringe driver pump) and an IV bag of glucose (via a volumetric pump). I cover continuous infusions in the later 'Administering Continuous Infusions: Insulin and Heparin' section and IV equipment in Chapter 14.

- **Intermittent infusion:** Drugs administered as a stat dose (immediately) or repeated over specific time intervals. These infusions are usually given over 15–20 minutes to 2 hours and are considered a compromise between a bolus injection and a continuous infusion. Volume amounts vary from 25–250 millilitres.

  When you're required to give two medications at the same time, for example, 1 litre sodium chloride 0.9% and a 100-millilitre bag with antibiotics added, this system is known as a *piggyback,* because the primary infusion and smaller secondary infusion can be administered together (as long as the infusions are compatible).

Examining electrolyte imbalances

Electrolytes are salts and minerals within the body, such as sodium, potassium and chloride, which can conduct electrical impulses in the body in order to maintain muscle function, bodily fluid amounts and the acidity of the arterial blood – which should be maintained within the pH range of 7.35 to 7.45.

Sensors detect and monitor the amount of electrolytes and water in the body. They're located within the body cells – in the *intracellular fluid* (ICF) – or outside of these cells – in the *extracellular fluid* (ECF). The concentration of electrolytes within the body is controlled by a variety of hormones mostly manufactured by the kidneys and the adrenal glands.

Hormones and electrolytes

The electrolyte balance is maintained within normal limits by the hormones, such as the following:

- ✔ Aldosterone (adrenal gland)
- ✔ Angiotensin (lung, brain and heart)
- ✔ Antidiuretic hormone (pituitary)
- ✔ Renin (kidneys)

Administering too-dilute or too-concentrated solutions can disrupt the balance of the electrolytes within the system, which is why hospital patients undergo blood testing to monitor these levels. Hypovolaemia (see Chapter 14) produces electrolyte disturbances that can affect the normal functioning of the nervous system, the heart and the kidneys; if prolonged it can result in acute renal failure.

Six important electrolytes

Electrolytes are *cations* (ions with a positive charge) or *anions* (ions with a negative charge). Here are the properties of six important electrolytes, along with their symptoms of excess and deficit and corrective treatment:

- ✔ **Sodium (Na+):** The major extracellular electrolyte. It influences water distribution in the body, because water goes where the sodium goes. Sodium also helps maintain fluid volume and plays a vital function in cellular activity, keeping the sodium in the plasma and the potassium inside the cell. Retention of sodium can result in fluid volume overload:

  - **Excess *(hypernatraemia):*** Observe for *polydipsia* (excessive thirst); dry, sticky mucous membranes; flushed skin and elevated temperature in first instance. Then watch for agitation, mental status changes, seizures and coma.

To correct hypernatraemia, restrict dietary sodium in first instance. Replace fluid volume with isotonic or slightly hypotonic saline if due to fluid loss.

- **Deficit *(hyponatraemia):*** Observe for nausea, headache, fatigue, tachycardia and vomiting in the first instance. More serious symptoms are confusion, muscle twitches, raised intracranial pressure, hemiparesis and seizures.

  To correct hyponatraemia, replace the sodium, orally in the first instance (by diet or supplement). If hyponatraemia is severe, administer hypertonic saline slowly in small amounts.

- **Normal serum levels:** 133–146 mmol/l.

✔ **Potassium (K+):** The most abundant intracellular electrolyte. It maintains equilibrium inside the cell and is influenced by changes in acid-base balance:

- **Excess *(hyperkalaemia):*** Observe for muscle weakness and in severe cases muscular flaccidity, peaked T-wave in ECG recordings, cardiac arrhythmias, including heart block and ventricular fibrillation. Hyperkalaemia is almost always associated with kidney disease and an inability to excrete enough (or any) potassium from the body.

  Correct hyperkalaemia with dietary restriction of potassium and review of medications, which may contain potassium. In severe cases, you can administer oral sodium polystyrene sulphonate.

- **Deficit *(hypokalaemia):*** Observe for constipation, fatigue, lethargy, muscle cramps, *parathesis* (numbness and tingling), diminished reflexes, cardiac arrhythmias and hypoventilation.

  To correct hypokalaemia, replace potassium by diet or oral supplements. You can treat severe hypokalaemia with slow IV therapy in a pre-mixed solution. Cardiac monitoring is recommended when administering potassium in higher concentrations.

  Never administer IV potassium by IV push; it can cause a cardiac arrest.

- **Normal serum levels:** 3.5–5.3 mmol/l.

✔ **Calcium (Ca²⁺):** Ninety-nine per cent of body calcium is found in teeth and bones, the rest being in extracellular fluid. Calcium is important for neuromuscular activity, normal cardiac electrophysiology, bone development and normal blood coagulation. When serum calcium levels drop below normal, the parathyroid gland secretes parathyroid hormone causing calcium to move from the bones into the blood.

The most common cause of low calcium in the body is due to not eating enough calcium rich foods and not getting enough vitamin D, which is necessary for intestinal absorption of calcium:

- **Excess** *(hypercalcaemia):* Observe for fatigue; gastrointestinal disturbances, such as nausea, vomiting and anorexia; weak and decreased tendon reflexes; confusion; *polyuria* (increased urination); cardiac complications such as decreased heart rate and arrhythmias; shortened QT interval; and atrioventricular (AV) block.

   Correct hypercalcaemia with hydration therapy orally or by IV therapy with normal saline. If the patient is hypervolaemic, an IV push of furosemide (loop diuretic) can accompany hydration therapy as a means of accelerating the excretion of calcium from the kidneys.

- **Deficit** *(hypocalcaemia):* Observe for general fatigue and muscle cramps in the first instance. As the condition progresses, check for parathesis, abdominal cramps, hyperactive tendon reflexes, *tetany* (muscle spasms and tremors), bronchospasm, seizures, cardiac arrhythmias (prolonged QT interval), congestive heart failure and shock.

   Correcting hypocalcaemia involves oral calcium supplements. In severe cases, IV therapy can include calcium gluconate or calcium chloride.

- **Normal serum levels:** Adjusted 2.2–2.6 mmol/l.

✔ **Magnesium (Mg2+):** Approximately 50–60 per cent of magnesium is found in the bones, the rest in the intracellular fluid. Magnesium is responsible for activating enzymes involved in the metabolism and for the proper functioning of nerves and muscles.

Patients at risk of low serum magnesium levels include malnourished patients, alcoholics, and patients with severe diarrhoea or those taking too high doses of diuretics:

- **Excess** *(hypermagnesaemia):* Observe for nausea, muscular problems, facial parathesis, respiratory depression, *bradycardia* (decreased respiratory rate) and cardiac arrest. Mild cases of hypermagnesaemia are asymptomatic, and so these are relatively late signs.

   Correct hypermagnesaemia by eliminating foods high in magnesium from the diet (tuna, artichokes, nuts) and conducting a medication review for any drugs high in this electrolyte. In severe cases, IV therapy may be initiated with calcium gluconate or for less severe cases with 0.45% normal saline.

- **Deficit** *(hypomagnesaemia):* Observe for parathesis, weakness, increased tendon reflexes, tetany, mild to severe mood changes, cardiac arrhythmias, seizures and ECG changes.

  Correct hypomagnesaemia through dietary or supplemental means. Severe cases may require IV therapy of magnesium sulphate in a diluted concentrate.

  When correcting hypomagnesaemia by IV therapy, you must observe the patient for magnesium toxicity; initially watch for a decrease in knee-jerk reflex, which disappears before respiratory depression (the most serious side effect of magnesium toxicity).

- **Normal serum levels:** 0.7–1.0 mmol/l.

✔ **Phosphate** (PO_4^{3-}): The major anion electrolyte. Phosphate is found mainly in the teeth and bones, but also in cells. Phosphorus occurs as phosphate and helps with acid-base balance, cellular energy metabolism and bone formation:

- **Excess** *(hyperphosphataemia):* Generally asymptomatic but may occur in conjunction with hypocalcaemia (see the earlier calcium bullet point).

  Correct hyperphosphataemia with IV normal saline in mild to moderate cases, and with intravenous calcium acetate in severe cases.

- **Deficit** *(hypophosphataemia):* Observe for vomiting, vitamin D deficiencies, hypercalcaemia, diabetic ketoacidosis, and alcoholism and patients withdrawing from alcohol.

  Correct hypophosphataemia by prevention. Doctors may advise patients to avoid taking medications that decrease phosphate levels in the blood. In severe cases, IV therapy may be initiated with sodium phosphate or potassium phosphate.

- **Normal serum levels:** 0.8–1.5 mmol/l.

✔ **Chloride (Cl–):** The most abundant extracellular electrolyte. Chloride is influenced by acid-base changes and is a component of the hydrochloric acid in the stomach.

Chloride and sodium imbalances often occur together:

- **Excess** *(hyperchloraemia):* Observe for symptoms of hypernatraemia (see the earlier sodium bullet point) in the first instance. In more severe cases, observe for *tachypnoea* (fast breathing rate), respiratory alkalosis and respiratory failure.

  Treat hyperchloraemia by correcting the primary electrolyte disturbance that caused it.

- **Deficit** *(hypochloraemia):* Observe for vomiting, diarrhoea, diuretics and patients drinking excessive amounts of water. Also observe for sweating, fever, increased muscular excitability, tetany, bradycardia and metabolic alkalosis.

  Treat hypochloraemia by correcting the primary electrolyte disturbance that caused it. If caused by hypovolaemia due to vomiting, replace the volume lost.

- **Normal serum levels:** 95–108 mmol/Ll.

Delivering Medications from Ampoules and Vials

You can draw up medications presented as liquids in vials and ampoules straight from the glass or plastic containers. Drugs presented in a freeze-dried powder format, however, need to have the medication *reconstituted,* which means adding liquid so that the medication can be administered via the IV route.

I show you how to reconstitute powdered medication and how to account for the 'displacement factor' – displacement what now?! Read on.

Knowing the correct way to reconstitute powdered medication

Most reconstituted medications require water for injection or sometimes saline. Some drugs require special diluents, which usually come with the drug in the packaging. To work out the dose, you use that most-useful of formula:

$$\frac{\text{What you want}}{\text{What you've got}} \times \text{Volume}$$

The volume amount is the amount of liquid you add to the ampoule to reconstitute. If you add 10 millilitres of water for injection to a 1,000 milligram ampoule, you notice that the total amount in your syringe is more than 10 millilitres. You have no problem here, though, because you're only after the total dose of the drug to be administered. However, if you have instructions to take into account the displacement factor, it's a different kettle of fish! Don't worry, check it out in the next section.

To prepare a drug from its powder form into a liquid form for IV drug administration, read the prescription chart and then follow these steps for the equilibrium method (this approach creates an equilibrium [state of balance] within the vial and helps to minimise the build-up of pressure in the vial):

1. **Wash hands, don apron and gather the following equipment: injection tray, medication ampoule, two syringe caps, diluent to reconstitute, non-sterile gloves, 0.9% sodium chloride for flush, two needles (one for the drug and one for the flush), two syringes (one for the drug and one for the flush), sharps container, two 70% alcohol and 2% chlorhexidine swabs (one for the ampoule and one for the access device).**

2. **Open the packaging and attach one of the needles to one of the syringes, put on the non-sterile gloves, protecting the key parts (the tip of the syringe and the hub of the needle).**

3. **Open the diluent and draw up the required volume.**

4. **Remove the lid from the ampoule, wipe the rubber seal with the swab in case of any contamination, for 30 seconds, and leave to dry for 30 seconds.**

5. **Insert the needle at an angle of 45–60 degrees into the ampoule.**

6. **Inject the correct amount of liquid slowly into the ampoule, keeping the tip of the needle above the level of the solution in the ampoule.**

7. **Release the plunger and the syringe should fill with air.**

8. **Hold the syringe and ampoule securely and agitate the contents gently, inspecting the contents to ensure that all medication has been dissolved.**

9. **Invert the ampoule, keeping the needle in the solution.**

10. **Inject air back into the ampoule by slowly depressing the plunger and then releasing it so that the solution flows back into the syringe.**

11. **Inject the diluent into the ampoule, keeping the tip of the needle above the level of the solution in the ampoule (then release the plunger and the syringe fills with air).**

12. **Withdraw the prescribed amount of solution and inspect the syringe to check that no pieces of rubber are inside.**

13. **Remove air from the syringe without spraying into the atmosphere by injecting the air back into the ampoule.**

14. **Replace sheath on needle by scooping up the sheath on the rigid injection tray, using one hand only in order to prevent needle-stick injuries, and adjust contents: that is, if prescription states 4.5 ml of drug to be administered, make sure that you have this amount in your syringe.**

15. **Expel any air from the syringe by tapping the syringe gently to remove any air bubbles.**

16. **Remove needle and cover the tip of syringe with a cap.**

17. **Label the syringe with the name of the drug inside.**

18. **Leave all equipment on the injection tray.**

19. **Draw up flush, protecting the key parts as above.**

20. **Label syringe and place in tray, after covering the tip of the syringe with the second cap.**

21. **Flush access site pre- and post-drug administration, after cleaning with 70% alcohol and 2% chlorhexidine swab, and put all sharps immediately in the sharps bin.**

22. **Document your actions.**

Accounting for the displacement factor

You may have heard about Archimedes, who (legend says) shouted 'Eureka!' when he worked out the principle of *displacement,* which in essence is the removal of one thing by something else taking its place.

You can test out his theory. Fill a bath to its fullest capacity and then get into the bath. Water splashes out all over your bathroom floor as your body raises the level of water in the bath. In this case, the displacement is the volume of your body occupying the volume that the fluid would otherwise occupy.

Now clean up the mess you made of your bathroom!

Many medications come in their ampoules freeze-dried ready for reconstitution. The manufacturer's instructions may ask you to reconstitute the drug with a certain amount of fluid. If so, you may need to apply the displacement factor.

Many healthcare areas use a form of injectable medicines administration guide to support areas administering medicines given via the intravenous subcutaneous and intramuscular routes. These guides give information in relation to the prescribing, dispensing and administration of these medicines (you can find one such guide at www.UCLHguide.com). Here are the procedural steps you need to undertake to reconstitute amoxicillin and taking into account the displacement factor.

Amoxicillin comes in vials of 250 and 500 milligrams:

1. **Add 5 ml of water for injection (WFI) to a 250 mg vial; add 10 ml of WFI to a 500 mg vial.**

2. **The injectable medicines guide states that the displacement value for the 250 mg vial is 0.2 ml and 0.4 ml for the 500 mg vial.**

   If using part of a vial, this means that you add only 4.8 ml to the 250 mg vial or 9.6 ml to the 500 mg vial, which gives a 50 mg/ml solution.

If you'd added 5 millilitres of WFI into the 250-milligram vial, you'd have been left with 5.2 millilitres of drug and infusate combined in your syringe. If you'd added 10 millilitres of WFI into a 500-millilgram vial, you'd have been left with 10.2 millilitres of drug and infusate combined in your syringe.

This next example shows you how to reconstitute another antibiotic taking into account a larger displacement factor. Piperacillin with tazobactam comes in vials of 2.25 and 4.5 grams:

1. **Add 10 ml of water for injection or normal saline for injection to a 2.25-g vial; add 20 ml of water for injection or normal saline to a 4.5g vial.**

2. **The injectable medicines guide states that the displacement value for the 2.25-g vial is 1.6 ml and 3.2 ml for the 4.5-g vial.**

   If using part of a vial, this means that you add only 8.4 ml water for injection or normal saline for injection to the 2.25-g vial, and 16.8 ml water for injection or normal saline to the 4.5-g vial. You then have a final concentration of 225 mg/ml.

As you can see, displacement comes into its own when using part of a vial or ampoule, but you need to know the basic principle. You may find that you'd only use part of a vial when the vial size is large and the prescribed amount is smaller.

Both amoxicillin and piperacillin with tazobactam are penicillins. Check allergy status before administration.

Now, I give you a chance to practise how this process may work in clinical practice. A small child weighing 6.80 kilograms (15 pounds) requires 340 milligrams of ceftazidime daily. You've been provided with a 2-gram vial, which needs to be reconstituted with WFI to make a total volume of 10 millilitres. The displacement value = 0.25 ml/250 mg.

Your task is to work out how many millilitres of WFI you need to add to the vial. Have a go yourself first and then carry on reading and see whether you're right!

You first note what size vial you have, in this case 2 grams (2,000 milligrams), and then work out the displacement value (250 mg/0.25 ml). You see that the 250 milligrams fits into the 2,000-milligram vial 8 times. This also equates to 8 lots of 0.25 ml WFI, which add up to 2 ml. Total volume = 10 ml minus the 2 ml = 8 millilitres of WFI to add to vial.

Therefore, you add 8 millilitres of WFI to the vial, leaving you with a total volume of 10 millilitres in the syringe, because the powder dissolved in the ampoule and took up room.

Being aware of drug administration timing considerations

You have to administer some drugs over a given time period, so as not to cause speed shock (which you can read about in Chapter 19).

This section explains how to work out the rate of these time-sensitive medicines. The rate of administration is in the administration guide of injectable medicines – www.UCLHguide.com – or in the manufacturer's information leaflet. Some of these drugs can be given as a bolus or by continuous infusion.

Here's the formula to use:

$$\text{Dose prescribed}\Big/\text{Rate}$$

Furosemide shouldn't exceed 4 milligrams of the drug over one minute. In this case, 20 milligrams of the drug is prescribed and drawn up. You put in the maximum dose per minute as the rate and use the formula as follows:

$$\frac{20 \text{ mg}}{4 \text{ mg}} = 5 \text{ minutes}$$

Therefore, you need to inject this drug over five minutes.

Here are some other IV drugs that need to be given over a set time period:

- **Aciclovir:** 250–500 mg (add to 100 ml bag normal saline [NS] for injection [sodium chloride] or glucose [G]). Rate: minimum of 1 hour.

- **Aminophylline:** 250 mg/10 ml (add required dose to 250 ml NS or G). Rate: over 20–30 minutes.

- **Amiodarone hydrochloride:** 5 mg/kg (add to 250 ml G). Rate: over 20 minutes to 2 hours.

- **Amoxicillin:** 250 mg with 5 ml WFI 500 mg with 10 ml WFI. Rate: over 3–4 minutes by bolus IV injection.

✔ **Diclofenac sodium (Voltarol brand):** 75 mg/3 ml. Dilute dose with 100–500 ml buffered NS or buffered G. To make the buffered infusion solution, add 0.5 ml sodium bicarbonate solution 8.4% to the bag before adding the diclofenac. Rate: 25–50 mg = over 15 minutes or longer; 75 mg = over 30 minutes or longer.

✔ **Omeprazole:** 40 mg reconstituted for IV bolus injection with 10 ml diluent (provided with drug). Rate: over 5 minutes.

Administering Continuous Infusions: Insulin and Heparin

You have to administer certain medications by *continuous infusion,* which means that the medication is given at a set rate over a period of time, but can be titrated according to medical condition by increasing or decreasing this rate. One example of a continuous infusion is patient-controlled analgesia (PCA). Here patients receive a combination of a set rate continuous background infusion and a supplementary bolus dose, which patients give themselves as required (see Chapter 14 for more on PCA).

Continuous infusions are usually indicated when constant blood levels are required, such as in the case of insulin and heparin IV administration (the focus of this section).

Use pre-prepared solutions where possible, such as heparin ampoules containing 20,000 units in 20 millilitres. Where a drug is to be mixed with a solution, you must mix it thoroughly so that the patient doesn't receive a too concentrated dose of the medication (known as precipitation or layering; see Chapter 19).

Infusing insulin

Blood glucose is the amount of glucose in the blood and is expressed as millimoles per litre of blood (mmol/l). Blood glucose levels vary throughout the day, before and after meals, but should stay within narrow parameters of 4–8 mmol/l (lowest in the morning and higher after meals).

Patients with Insulin Dependent Diabetes Mellitus (IDDM) require insulin injections, which can be as follows:

✔ **Short acting:** For example, actrapid (lasts for no more than 8 hours).

✔ **Intermediate acting:** For example, insulatard (lasts 12–24 hours).

✔ **Long acting:** For example, ultratard (lasts 24–36 hours).

Blood glucose levels

Normal blood glucose levels tend to remain between 4 and 8 mmols/l, though in cardiopulmonary resuscitation a reading of 4–10 mmol/l is often the acceptable range. Glucose levels vary from person to person, but a blood sugar level of 50 milligrams per decilitre (mg/dl) or less is considered to be *hypoglycaemic*. Just a note, a decilitre is equal to one tenth of a litre.

In contrast, *hyperglycaemia* is where the blood glucose levels are considered excessively high.

It occurs when the body doesn't have enough insulin or is unable to turn this insulin within the body into energy. Hyperglycaemia is often an indicator of out-of-control diabetes mellitus.

Insulin was originally an extract of pig or bovine pancreas. Today, human insulin is made in the laboratory by combining the human gene that codes for insulin with the genetic material of bacteria or yeasts.

Patients can acquire their insulin via an intermittent infusion when they come into the hospital situation, which can be titrated according to their blood glucose readings, and is usually monitored hourly (a sliding scale).

The protocol for IV insulin therapy varies from hospital to hospital, but a usual prescription is to administer a second intravenous infusion of 0.9% sodium chloride or 5% glucose, depending on the blood glucose readings. These infusions run simultaneously. Infusion 1 (insulin – usually administered via a syringe driver pump) and Infusion 2 (saline or glucose – usually administered via a volumetric pump) are connected using a Y connector device containing the two non-return valves, which are connected to the same cannula (see Figure 15-1).

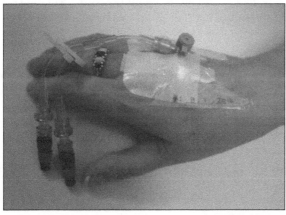

Figure 15-1:
Cannula
with Y
connector
attached.

© John Wiley & Sons, Inc.

Infusion 1 is usually made up of 50 units actrapid (0.5 ml of 100 units/ml drawn up in an insulin syringe):

1. **Add the 50 units of actrapid to sodium chloride 0.9% to make a total volume of 50 ml (this means that you add only 49.5 ml to the syringe, and then add the actrapid [0.5 ml] to make a total of 50 ml in a Luer Lock syringe and thoroughly mix).**

2. **Add an extension line to the end of the Luer Lock syringe and prime.**

3. **Flush the patient's cannula after cleaning to check its *patency* (that the line is clear and not obstructed), and then attach the end of the extension line to the patient's Y connector (attached to the patient's cannula).**

4. **Set up the Luer Lock syringe in the appropriate infusion pump.**

Some syringe drivers are designed to accept 20-millilitre infusions in 20-millilitre Luer Lock syringes. In all cases, attach a label to the syringe stating the contents of the syringe in the syringe driver, making sure not to cover the graduations on the syringe.

Infusion 2 (0.9% sodium chloride or 5% glucose) is set up via an IV adminis-tration set and volumetric pump and attached to the Y connector.

You can then start Infusions 1 and 2. Measure the blood glucose hourly, adjusting the sliding scale insulin according to local protocol and recording using the correct documentation. If the insulin infusion is commenced on your diabetic patient because she's going for surgery, set an adult syringe driver at 2–4 units/hr and a child's at 0.5 units/kg/hr.

A usual initial infusion rate for adults in a diabetic emergency, known as *dia-betic ketoacidosis,* is 6 units administered as an IV bolus injection, followed by 6 units by infusion.

Pump observations, like a fluid chart, should record a 'running total', which is a record of the amount of units or millilitres a patient has received over a set period of time.

An insulin infusion containing 50 international units (IU) of human actrapid has been diluted with 50 millilitres of sodium chloride. You're asked to work out how many units of actrapid insulin in total the patient has received.

To find the answer, you add up the rates, which in this case are as follows:

✔ 3 ml/hr for 2 hours = 6.0 ml

✔ 3.5 ml/ hr for 3 hours = 10.5 ml

- ✔ 2 ml/hr for 1 hour = 2.0 ml
- ✔ 2.5 ml/hr for 1 hour = 2.5 ml
- ✔ 4 ml/hr for 2 hours = 8.0 ml

50 units = 50 millilitres (the ratio is 1:1) and so the patient has received 29.0 units of actrapid over 9 hours.

Handling heparin infusions

Heparin is from a class of drugs known as anticoagulants and is often prescribed to prevent blood clots from forming in the veins, arteries or lungs, or to treat existing blood clots in the blood vessels from getting any larger. Unfractionated heparin is available in varying strengths, such as the following:

- ✔ **1,000 units/ml:** In ampoules or vials of 1ml, 5ml, 10 ml, 20 ml
- ✔ **5,000 units/ml:** In ampoules or vials of 1ml, 5 ml
- ✔ **20,000 units/20 ml:** In vials of 20 ml
- ✔ **25,000 units/ml:** In ampoules or vials of 1 ml, 5 ml

Unfractionated heparin and low-molecular-weight heparin (for example, enoxaparin and tinzaparin) differ from each other according to the size and weight of the heparin molecules (see Chapter 5 for more details).

Heparin works by decreasing the clotting ability of the blood. The activated partial thromboplastin time (APTT) is a common laboratory test that measures the clotting time by checking how long the blood takes to clot (in seconds). In short, the APTT test checks that the blood contains enough heparin to prevent clotting, but not so much as to cause bleeding.

Therefore, before starting a heparin infusion, you need to measure the patient's baseline APPT by sending a sample of her blood to the laboratory for this reading. The greater the APTT value, the longer the blood takes to clot: high APTT equals a risk of bleeding and low APTT equals a risk of blood clots/stroke.

You administer heparin IV therapy to patients via a syringe driver pump (see Chapter 14). Different hospitals have their own protocol for intravenous heparin infusions, with many requesting a baseline platelet count, as well as the baseline APTT. A typical protocol may then require the patient first to have a 'loading dose' of heparin IV administered, such as: 5,000 units (5 ml of heparin solution 1,000 units/ml) bolus IV over 3–5 minutes.

The initial infusion rate is then titrated according to weight in kilograms (18 units/kg/hr), as I show in Table 15-1.

Table 15-1	Heparin Rates According to Body Weight
Weight in Kg	*Initial Infusion Rate*
40–49	0.8 ml (800 units) per hour
50–59	1.0 ml (1,000 units) per hour
60–69	1.1 ml (1,100 units) per hour
70–79	1.2 ml (1,200 units) per hour
80–89	1.4 ml (1,400 units) per hour
90–99	1.6 ml (1,600 units) per hour
100–109	1.8 ml (1,800 units) per hour
110–119	2.0 ml (2,000 units) per hour
120–129	2.2 ml (2,200 units) per hour
130 and over	2.4 ml (2,400 units) per hour

Using the numbers in the table, you can discern the necessary infusion rate settings for different patients. For example:

- ✔ A patient weighing 52 kg needs the initial infusion rate set at 1.0 ml per hour.

- ✔ A patient weighing 80 kg needs the initial infusion rate set at 1.4 ml per hour.

- ✔ A patient weighing 112 kg needs the initial infusion rate set at 2.0 ml per hour.

You place the heparin in the syringe driver pump and prepare it by drawing up the contents of an ampoule containing 20,000 units in 20 ml, and setting the pump to run at the required infusion rate, as per Table 15-1.

Check the APTT six hours after starting the infusion – to find what's called the *APTT ratio* – using the following formula:

$$\text{APTT ratio} = \frac{\text{Latest APTT}}{\text{Baseline APTT}}$$

A patient's baseline APTT was recorded as 23 seconds. Six hours after starting the infusion, her APTT is 30.6 seconds. You calculate her APTT ratio as follows:

$$\frac{30.6 \text{ seconds}}{23 \text{ seconds}} = 1.33 \text{ seconds}$$

After obtaining the APTT ratio, you adjust the infusion rate as per Table 15-2.

Table 15-2	Activated Partial Thromboplastin Time (APTT) Ratio Infusion Rates	
APTT Ratio (Seconds)	**Action**	**Recheck APTT Ratio After:**
Less than 1.2	Increase rate by 0.4 ml (400 units) per hour. Additional 5,000 units bolus to be prescribed on in-patient chart	6 hours (urgent priority)
1.2 – 1.49	Increase rate by 0.2 ml (200 units) per hour	6 hours (urgent priority)
1.5 – 2.5	No change	24 hours
2.51 – 3	Reduce rate by 0.1 ml (100 units) per hour	6 hours (urgent priority)
3.01 – 4	Reduce rate by 0.3 ml (300 units) per hour	6 hours (urgent priority)
More than 4	Stop infusion for 1 hour and then reduce rate by 0.5 ml (500 units) per hour	6 hours (urgent priority)

If APTT is less than 1.2 or greater than 4, inform medical staff and document actions in the medical notes.

Heparin can cause hyperkalaemia (see the earlier section 'Examining electrolyte imbalances'). Measure the plasma potassium in patients at risk before starting heparin therapy and in all patients treated for more than seven days. Also, measure the patient's platelet count on the day following heparin commencement for all patients who've been exposed to heparin in the last 100 days, and on alternate days from days 4 to 14 for all patients.

An adult unfractionated heparin intravenous infusion has been running for six hours at 0.8 millilitres per hour (800 units). The heparin infusion is made up as 20,000 units in 20 millilitres.

First, how many millilitres of the drug has the patient received?

To find the answer, multiple 0.8 millilitres by 6 hours to get 4.8 millilitres (4,800 units, but you don't need to give this information because the question doesn't ask for it).

Second, the rate is changed for the next six hours, decreasing the initial rate by 0.2 ml. What's the total amount that the patient has received now (in 12 hours)?

You take the current rate (0.8 ml – 0.2 ml = 0.6 ml) and multiple by 6 hours, which gives 3.6 ml (over 6 hours). You then add 4.8 ml (over the first 6 hours) for a grand total of 8.4 ml (over 12 hours).

Chapter 16

Round Peg in a Square Hole: Getting Drugs and Fluids into the Body

*Y*ou're standing next to a patient who needs some fluids or liquid medication. You can't just pour it into a cup and ask him to drink it, because it has to be released gradually into his system. To get medications and fluids in through the intravenous (IV) route, you require an access device (please don't try it without one – messy!). The umbrella term for these devices is a *vascular access device* (VAD).

This chapter looks at the different types of available access devices, how to use them and the problems that can arise. Some of these devices are left in place for a few days and are considered short term, whereas others are longer term, staying in place for weeks or months.

When administering drugs and/or fluids into VADs, always maintain a strict aseptic approach, known as the aseptic and aseptic non-touch technique (ANTT), to prevent infections.

Introducing IV Access Devices

When selecting the appropriate access device for IV therapy, you need to undertake a full assessment of the patient's requirements to decide whether a short-term or longer-term device is required.

Popping in for a few days: Peripheral cannulae

The usual method for IV therapy is to use what's commonly called a *peripheral cannula* (or more fully a *peripheral vascular access device*), which is often sited in the hand or arm. These devices are usually left in place for a period of about three days, and so are considered short-term access devices. I cover this type of device in the later section 'Going for the Vein: Peripheral Cannulae'.

The most common veins used for this system are as follows:

- **Basilic vein:** Wrist area of arm

- **Cephalic vein:** Just above wrist area of arm

- **Dorsal venous network:** Back of hand

Refer to Figure 16-1 for an illustration of veins used for inserting peripheral cannulae.

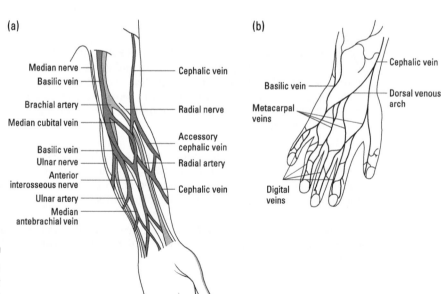

(a)

Median nerve
Basilic vein
Brachial artery
Median cubital vein
Basilic vein
Ulnar nerve
Anterior interosseous nerve
Ulnar artery
Median antebrachial vein

Cephalic vein
Radial nerve
Accessory cephalic vein
Radial artery
Cephalic vein

(b)

Cephalic vein
Basilic vein
Dorsal venous arch
Metacarpal veins
Digital veins

Figure 16-1: Veins for inserting peripheral cannulae.

© *John Wiley & Sons, Inc.*

Staying for the longer haul: Central lines

Other devices used for IV therapy, usually in the longer term (weeks and months), are central lines (or central venous access devices [CVAD]), with the lines being of variable lengths according to the type.

Central lines are placed in the larger central veins of the body. Before infusing through a newly placed central line, the device's tip location needs to be confirmed with a chest X-ray.

Many central line devices are available. Peripherally inserted central catheters (known as PICC lines) are a specific type of central line, which tend to be used for patients requiring several weeks or months of IV therapy. Other less common devices that you may encounter include the following:

- ✔ **Short-term percutaneous central venous catheter (CVC) (non-tunnelled):** For patients requiring just days or weeks of IV access.
- ✔ **Skin-tunnelled catheters:** For patients requiring long-term IV access. These lines are often called 'wiggles' by children.
- ✔ **Implantable ports:** For patients requiring long-term IV access.

I discuss central lines in detail in the later 'Getting Drugs into the Central System' section. The medical practitioner decides which access device is most suitable for the patient's condition.

Going for the Vein: Peripheral Cannulae

A *peripheral cannula* is the most common IV access device used in the healthcare setting. The needle of the device locates the vein and the plastic cannula then slips over the needle to sit in the vein. You then discard the needle into a sharps bin.

I cover all aspects of using a peripheral cannula in this section.

Introducing peripheral cannulae

The veins used for peripheral cannulae tend to be those located in the hand and lower arm. To a much lesser degree, these devices can be sited in the leg and foot. In infants, the scalp veins are sometimes used.

Applying access devices to legs, feet and scalps may require extra training, because not all healthcare professionals are permitted to use these sites. Using the lower extremities in adults isn't recommended due to the risk of embolism and thrombophlebitis.

After siting the device, secure it in place – with some type of stabilisation device – and cover with a sterile dressing (transparent or low-linting gauze). Figure 16-2 shows a cannula secured in place with tapes, covered with a dressing and an IV drip attachment being connected.

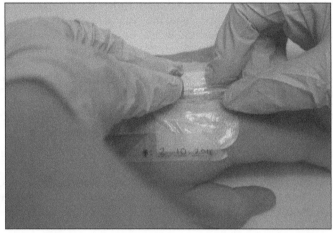

Figure 16-2:
A secured
cannula.

© John Wiley & Sons, Inc.

Gauging the cannula size

Peripheral cannulae come in different gauge sizes: for example, 14 gauge (14 G) is large and often used in resuscitation settings to get emergency drugs into the body quickly, whereas gauges 24–26 are the smallest size.

Table 16-1 shows which gauge size to choose on patients, along with the common applications and flow rates of IV fluids (in litres per hour). For example, different cannulae, depending on their size, allow the fluids to be delivered into the vein at different rates – the larger the cannula size, the quicker the rate of fluid into the body. The table shows that a 20-gauge cannula can deliver 1.9 litres of blood into the body, per hour.

Choosing the most appropriate gauge size for paediatric patients is established after assessing the veins and selecting the most appropriate site and after obtaining the child's weight and age. Table 16-2 shows the general gauge sizes depending on age.

Table 16-1 Peripheral Cannulae Gauges and Flow Rates

Gauge Size	Common Application	Approx. Flow Rate (L/hour): Crystalloid	Approx. Flow Rate (L/hour): Plasma	Approx. Flow Rate (L/hour): Blood
14 G	In theatres or emergencies for rapid transfusion of blood or viscous fluids	16.2	13.5	10.3
16 G	In theatres or emergencies for rapid transfusion of blood or viscous fluid	10.8	9.4	7.1
17 G	Blood transfusions; rapid infusion of large volumes of viscous liquids	7.5	6.5	4.6
18 G	Blood transfusions; parenteral nutrition; stem cell harvesting and cell separation; large volumes of fluids	4.8	4.1	2.7
20 G	Blood transfusions; large volumes of fluids	3.2	2.9	1.9
22 G	Blood transfusions; most medications and fluids	1.9	1.7	1.1
24 G	Medications, short-term infusions; fragile veins; children	0.8	0.7	0.5
26 G	Neonatal (see Table 16-2 for details)	0.8	0.7	0.5

Table 16-2 Cannula Gauge Sizes for Children

Age of Child	Weight in Kilograms	Peripheral IV Gauge
Premature infant	3 or less	26–22
Neonate	3–4	26–22
1 month to 11 months	4–10	24–20
1 year to 2 years	10–13	24–20
3 years to 5 years	13–18	24–20
6 years to 12 years	18–40	24–18
Adolescent aged 13 to 18 years	40–75	24–18

Making the job easier

To make the insertion of the cannula less painful for children, or for patients with needle phobias, you can apply a topical local anaesthetic to the insertion area to numb the site for about 30–60 minutes beforehand. More specifically, consider using a topical anaesthetic in the following situations:

- ✔ Anxious patients
- ✔ Patient request
- ✔ Using a sensitive area, such as the wrist
- ✔ Using a large device, such as 18 G or larger

You apply the anaesthetic cream to at least two sites, cover with transparent dressing and wait the recommended time for the medication to work. Here are the instructions for two commonly used creams/gels:

- ✔ **EMLA:** Apply 60 minutes prior to cannulation. Side effects to watch for include vasoconstriction.
- ✔ **AMETOP:** Apply 30 minutes (but no longer than 45) prior to cannulation. Side effects to watch for include erythematous rash and itching.

These topical anaesthetics also come in a spray format.

A peripheral cannula can be used for only a short period of time, usually three days, before being replaced. Otherwise, bacteria on the skin can travel into the bloodstream or surrounding tissue and cause bacterial phlebitis (see the later 'Checking for problems' section), cellulitis and sepsis.

You administer the medication by the hub (situated at the top of the device, covered by the cap) or more usually from an extension line at the end of the device. These devices require *priming:* that is, filling with saline prior to insertion to remove the air (see Chapter 14 for details).

Figure 16-3 shows a double lumen extension line: lumen is Latin for an opening – therefore a double lumen is having two openings or ports of entry.

The device then requires regular flushing, using a 5-millilitre – or preferably larger 10-millilitre – syringe, to maintain *patency* (keeping the cannula clear and unobstructed) and before and after each use, using 0.9% sodium chloride. This is because using a smaller syringe increases the pressure, which has the potential to damage the intima of the vein.

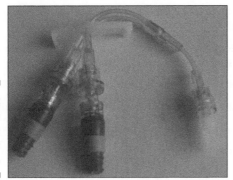

Figure 16-3: Double lumen extension line.

Use a push-pause motion while flushing (often referred to as a 'stop-start' technique) so that you create turbulence to remove debris from the internal catheter. Inspect the site regularly and record all information in the patient's care plan and/or notes.

Inserting a peripheral cannulae

After training, the procedure for inserting a peripheral cannula is relatively simple, as long as you adhere to key principles, such as infection control and the aseptic and aseptic non-touch technique.

Different clinical areas can have their own procedural steps, but in general the process is along the following lines:

1. **Introduce yourself to the patient, explain the procedure, gain consent, invite questions and check the patient's medical history and any medication he's taking.**

   Apply topical anaesthetic, if required (and wait for the anaesthetic to work); see the preceding section for details.

2. **Assemble all the equipment required, checking all packaging and looking for damaged or out-of-date equipment.**

   Here's what you need: sterile dressing pack, cannulae of varying gauge sizes, alcohol hand-rub, chloraprep swab (or similar skin-cleaning equipment), extension line, non-sterile gloves and apron, cannula dressing, 5–10 ml syringe, 21 G needle, 0.9% sodium chloride 5–10 ml ampoule, single patient use tourniquet, injection tray with sharps container.

3. **Wash hands using soap and water.**

   Return to the bedside.

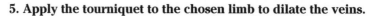

4. Get patient into a comfortable position, preferably on a bed with chosen limb on a pillow.

Check height of bed for your comfort. Check for good light source and privacy. Decontaminate hands using alcohol hand-rub.

5. Apply the tourniquet to the chosen limb to dilate the veins.

Assess and select the vein you want to use. Release the tourniquet.

You have six ways of encouraging veins to dilate:

- Using a tourniquet
- Letting gravity do its work by lowering the arm below heart level, which also increases blood supply to the veins
- Opening and closing the fist (the patient's not yours, no matter how nervous you are!)
- Stroking/gentle rubbing the vein
- Heating by, for example, immersing the arm in a bowl of warm water for 10 minutes to encourage vasodilation and venous filling
- Using ointment or patches containing small amounts of glyceryl trinitrate to cause local vasodilation to aid venepuncture

6. Select the cannula device based on the vein size.

Clean the patient's skin around the area of the selected vein site for 30 seconds using the chloraprep swab (or similar). Leave to dry for 30 seconds.

Don't re-palpate the vein or touch the skin again after cleaning.

7. Wash hands using soap and water or alcohol hand-rub and put on gloves and apron.

Open dressing pack, empty all equipment onto pack and place a sterile dressing towel under the patient's arm. Re-apply the tourniquet.

Although many clinical areas now consider that best practice is to use a sterile dressing pack when inserting a peripheral cannula, others prefer to use an aseptic non-touch technique (ANTT).

8. Inspect the cannula for any faults.

Anchor the vein by applying manual traction on the skin a few centimetres below the proposed site of insertion and where you've cleaned the skin. Ensure that the cannula bevel is in the upright position and place the device directly over the vein; insert the cannula through the skin at the selected angle according to the depth of the vein. Wait for the flashback of blood that you can see in the chamber of the stylet.

9. **Level the device by decreasing the angle between the cannula and the skin and advance the cannula slightly to ensure entry into the lumen of the vein.**

   Withdraw the stylet slightly and watch for the second flashback of blood along the shaft of the cannula.

10. **Maintain skin traction with your non-dominant hand and using your dominant hand slowly advance the cannula off the stylet and into the vein.**

    Release the tourniquet.

11. **Apply digital pressure to the vein above the cannula tip and remove the stylet.**

    Dispose of stylet immediately into the sharps container.

12. **Attach an extension line (or IV drip administration line or other) to the cannula.**

    Secure the cannula with tapes from the sterile dressing pack. Flush the cannula with sodium chloride 0.9% using the push-pause technique (from the preceding section).

13. **Observe the site for signs of swelling or leakage and ask the patient whether he feels any discomfort or pain.**

    If so, you may need to remove the cannula and resite in a different position. The key point is always to listen to your patient. Cover the cannula with the dressing.

14. **Discard waste.**

    Remove apron and gloves and wash hands with soap and water. Document the date and time of insertion, site and size of cannula in the patient's notes and care plan (containing the visual inspection of phlebitis assessment; see the next section).

Voilà! You now have access to the IV route and can use it for drug administration.

Checking for problems

Table 16-3 shows a few trouble-shooting tips for when you're inserting a peripheral cannula, with actions to overcome any difficulties.

Visual Infusion Phlebitis (known as the VIP score) is the assessment of the cannula site, observing for any signs of pain and redness. The VIP score involves observing the access device insertion site and arm for any signs of infection. I discuss the VIP assessment in more depth in Chapter 18.

Table 16-3	Factors Affecting Cannulation Insertion and Actions to Resolve the Situation	
Patient Details	**Why This Affects the Clinical Skill of Cannulation**	**Action**
Patient with a right-sided cerebral vascular accident (stroke)	Using the left arm/hand may further reduce the patient's ability to perform activities of living. In turn, using this arm/hand can result in poor access due to the veins in this non-affected arm being used all the time. Also, the arm/hand of the affected side may have loss of sensation and if you cause damage to a nerve, the patient may not be able to feel and express the pain.	Locate the cannula away from joints to prevent restriction of movement.
Patient following mastectomy and axillary lymph node dissection	Only has one arm available for use due to the surgery. If you use the arm on the side of the mastectomy and axillary lymph node dissection, putting on a tourniquet increases the risk of lymphoedema occurring. Because the veins in the arm unaffected by the surgery are used all the time, this can result in poor access.	Use smallest device possible to do the least amount of damage and ensure good aseptic technique to prevent any risk of infection. Cannulate on the opposite side of surgery, if able. Avoid cannulating over joints that would prevent restriction of movement.
Anxious or needle-phobic patient	If they have prior adverse outcomes or experiences, or a dislike of medical procedures.	Listen to the person's experiences and concerns. Offer privacy, an opportunity to lie/sit in a comfortable position, social support and local anaesthetic. Explaining procedure, where appropriate showing equipment, and involving the patient in the choice of vein, can increase a feeling of control and help relieve anxiety. Give information on the need for the blood tests/cannula insertion and length of time the procedure will take. Be confident, efficient and successful first time. Distraction is a useful technique for the mildly anxious patient, for example, asking the patient to cough while simultaneously undertaking the venepuncture/cannula insertion.

Patient Details	Why This Affects the Clinical Skill of Cannulation	Action
Patient who speaks no English or can't communicate easily	Unable to get verbal consent; failure to get valid consent can be viewed as physical assault on a patient as well as being disrespectful and unprofessional. Unable to confirm details verbally, establish any prior problems with these procedures or determine the patient's understanding of the procedure and necessity of the blood test/cannula insertion. Possible complications need to be explained to the patient.	Check identification band. Use interpreter or member of family if available. Use language line or similar interpreting service provider, if appropriate. Don't take blood if you can't identify the patient and/or feel that the patient doesn't fully understand the procedure and therefore hasn't given consent.
Patient who has refused the procedure	Verbal consent is required. Failure to seek valid consent can be viewed as physical assault on a patient as well as being disrespectful and unprofessional. Consent needs to be voluntary and given without influence or undue pressure to accept or refuse the treatment. Possible complications and the reason for having blood taken/device inserted need to be fully explained to the patient.	Ask the patient why he's refusing the procedure using appropriate questioning technique. Effective communication and discussion should be documented in the patient notes and the doctors informed of the patient's refusal to the procedure.
Patient on anticoagulation therapy	Risk of prolonged bleeding time post-procedure and risk of haematoma formation	Ascertain patient's current International Normalised Ratio (INR; see Chapter 11) status if possible. Use smallest device possible and apply tourniquet for as short a time as possible. Apply pressure on site and check that site has stopped bleeding before leaving patient. If bruising occurs, inform patient and explain what can be done to reduce it. Monitor the site and provide reassurance. If a haematoma forms, apply pressure and inform appropriate medical/nursing staff. Ensure that patient understands that he should report if any numbness occurs (indicating pressure on nerve) and when to report back to the hospital, and document it.

(continued)

Table 16-3 *(continued)*

Patient Details	Why This Affects the Clinical Skill of Cannulation	Action
Types of vein to avoid when selecting a site for cannulation	*Thrombosed and hard:* painful for patient; increased damage to vein. *Inflamed:* painful for patient; can increase risk of infection. *Thin/fragile:* bruise easily; increased risk of infiltration/ extravasation. *Bruised:* cannulation likely to be unsuccessful, painful for patient. *Mobile:* harder to anchor and therefore risk of unsuccessful cannulation. *Tortuous:* may not be able to advance the length of cannula. *Multiple punctures:* painful for patient; risk of infiltration/ extravasation; increased injury to vessel. *Near bones and over joint:* movement of joint causes painful and discomfort for the patient. *Infection:* increased risk of infection; avoid veins adjacent to the foci of infection due to risk of causing more local tissue damage or systemic infection. *Oedemas:* avoid oedematous areas due to danger of stasis of lymph; causes pain for the patient.	Spend time selecting an appropriate vein.

Securing and dressing the access site

You need to secure the cannula in place with a sterile dressing, ensuring that it allows clear visibility of the insertion site for inspection. If the dressing becomes loose or soiled, change using an aseptic technique.

You can apply a secondary dressing, using a correctly sized Tubifast or bandage, to protect the cannula from inadvertently being knocked out – for instance, in the case of paediatric nursing or with confused patients. You have to remove these covers when observing the insertion of the cannula sites in their entirety to be able to truly view for any signs of infection.

You can use non-sterile tape to support the administration set/weight of lines, but *don't* secure to the cannula dressing. You've been told!

Sampling blood from the cannula

You can sample blood from a cannula only immediately following insertion, unless the patient has such poor veins that you can't readily obtain a sample from another site.

If a blood sample is to be obtained via a pre-existing cannula, you must discard the first 5 millilitres in adults (less in children depending on their age and size) and flush the cannula after the procedure with 5–10 millilitres of 0.9% sodium chloride.

Removing the cannula

When the cannula is removed, check that it's complete – in other words, that no part of the device has broken off and been left inside the patient's vein. If you have any suspicion that the cannula is incomplete, contact the patient's medical team.

When removing a cannula, you ideally must use a sterile dressing, such as gauze, to apply pressure and dress the site. Wear gloves and apron for the removal procedure. Make sure that you document the removal of the cannula in the appropriate patient record.

Getting Drugs into the Central System

Central lines (or central venous access devices – CVADs) are access devices placed into the larger veins, usually in the superior vena cava or inferior vena cava through the neck or within the right atrium of the heart through the chest wall.

Depending on the type of central line, a medical practitioner performs the procedure, with a nurse assisting. Specialist nurses can insert devices, such as a Groshong line – a specific type of skin-tunnel device often used for chemotherapy. A portacath is always conducted by medical staff, because it's a surgical procedure. Figure 16-4 shows where the central line is placed.

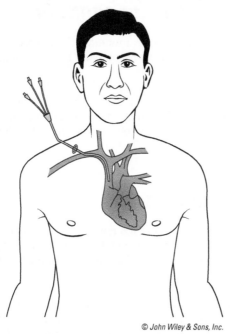

Figure 16-4:
Central line
placement.

© John Wiley & Sons, Inc.

These sections provide a clearer picture of what you need to know when inserting a central line.

Riding the central line

In the simplest type of central line, a catheter is inserted into the subclavian, internal jugular or (less commonly) a femoral vein and advanced towards the heart until it reaches the superior vena cava or right atrium. After insertion of the catheter, a chest X-ray is performed to check that the line has been sited in the correct position and to rule out the occurrence of *pneumothorax* (air or gas in the pleural cavity), *haemothorax* (blood in the pleural cavity) or cardiac tamponade (see the nearby 'Dangerous pressure on the heart' sidebar). Figure 16-5 shows a selection of central lines.

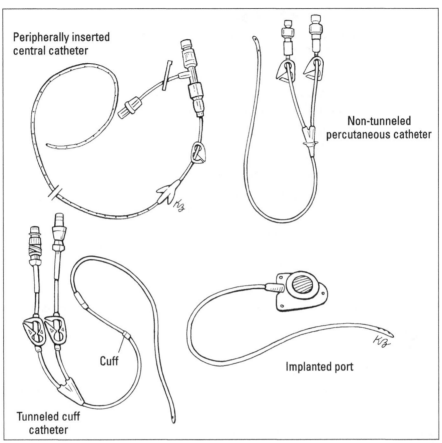

Peripherally inserted central catheter

Non-tunneled percutaneous catheter

Cuff

Tunneled cuff catheter

Implanted port

Figure 16-5: A selection of central lines.

Illustration by Kathyrn Born

TECHNICAL STUFF

Dangerous pressure on the heart

Cardiac tamponade is a serious medical condition in which blood or fluid fill the space between the sac that encases the heart and the heart muscle. This fluid puts extreme pressure on the heart, preventing the heart's ventricles from expanding fully and functioning properly. As a result, not enough blood is pumped to the rest of the body, which can lead to organ failure, shock and possibly death.

Identifying advantages of central lines

Central lines have several advantages over the peripheral cannulae that I discuss earlier in 'Going for the Vein: Peripheral Cannulae':

- ✔ Central lines go into veins that carry blood directly into the heart so medication is more quickly distributed to the rest of the body, which is essential in emergency resuscitation situations, for example.

- ✔ Central lines can deliver fluids and medications that cause irritation to peripheral veins due to their concentration or chemical composition, including chemotherapy drugs, extended antibiotic regimes and some kinds of parenteral nutrition.

- ✔ Health professionals can use central lines to measure central venous pressure and other physical variables through the line.

- ✔ Central lines provide room for multiple applications of medications using double or triple lumen devices – meaning two, three or more lines in one device.

Some drugs and solutions are hypotonic/hypertonic and should only administered by a central line, because given peripherally they can damage the vain: concentrated potassium fluids, dextrose 20%/dextrose 50%, dobutamine, dopamine, ganciclovir, metraminol and noradrenalin among others.

Considering the risks to central lines

Central lines do carry more risks than peripheral cannulae, however, and are more difficult to insert correctly. Therefore, they require experienced, skilled staff to safely locate and enter the vein correctly. The nurse's role is usually to assist the medical team during the procedure.

Here are the main risks to central lines:

- ✔ **Air embolism:** The risk of getting air into the venous system is much higher with a central line device on insertion, and can also occur up to 48 hours after removal of the line. All connections need to be clamped off when not in use to prevent air entry, and the lines primed with fluid before connection. A large pulmonary air embolus can cause death by blocking the vein and stopping the heart.

- ✔ **Bleeding:** Arterial puncture caused by accidently puncturing the carotid, vertebral, subclavian, basilic, axillary or femoral arteries on insertion.

- ✔ **Cardiac dysrhythmias:** Occur if the catheter tip touches the cardiac wall, affecting the rate and rhythm of the heart due to 'tickling' the sino atrial node – the peacemaker of the heart.

- ✔ **Infection:** As the line goes directly to the heart, bacterial contamination can be quickly spread throughout the body, resulting in septicaemia.

- ✔ **Misdirection:** Or 'kinking' of the line can occlude the adminis-tered fluids.

- ✔ **Pinch off syndrome**: Where the central line is compressed between the first rib and the clavicle, causing an infusion occlusion in subclavian vein inserted CVAD.

- ✔ **Pneumothorax:** Can occur if the catheter punctures the chest wall and allows air to enter the pleural cavity.

Taking a look at other central lines

Central lines come in different types – but all are long, hollow tubes with the tip sited into a large vein just above the heart, with the other end coming out of the chest and sealed with a cap or bung through which the medication or infusion is administered. This section describes four types of central lines.

The general time limits for central lines are as follows:

- ✔ **Less than 10 days:** Non-tunnelled central venous catheter (CVC), PICC or midline devices

- ✔ **10 days to 4 weeks:** PICC or midline devices

- ✔ **4 weeks to 6 months:** PICC, tunnelled CVC or totally implantable vascu-lar access devices (TIVAD, known as ports or portacaths)

- ✔ **6 months, up to 6 years:** Tunnelled CVC or TIVAD devices

Peripherally inserted central catheters (PICC lines)

A PICC line is a special type of central line. You insert the cannula through a peripheral vein (usually in the axilla or the antecubital fossa – the bit that bends in the arm!) and edge the tip of the cannula slowly upwards until it's in a central vein.

This type of device is used for patients requiring medication therapy, such as chemotherapy, renal interventions and so on, because the lines can be left in place for weeks or months. Refer to Figure 16-6 for where a PICC line is placed.

Short-term percutaneous central venous catheters (non-tunnelled)

These devices go through the skin directly into a central vein and are used for therapy that may last from a few days to several weeks.

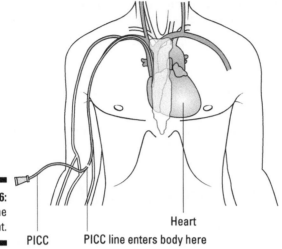

Figure 16-6:
A PICC line
placement.

PICC   PICC line enters body here   Heart

© John Wiley & Sons, Inc.

They can be used for emergency fluid replacement and for central venous pressure readings and where the patient has an absence of peripheral veins.

Skin-tunnelled catheters

These catheters are long-term devices that lie in a subcutaneous tunnel (between the sternum and the nipple) in order to enter a central vein – usually subclavian, or jugular, axillary or femoral, with the tip of the line usually placed at the superior vena cava junction.

These devices are used when peripheral vascular access is problematic.

Implantable ports

These systems are implanted vascular devices comprising two components – a reservoir attached to a catheter – inserted on the chest or arm in order to reach the antecubital fossa, subclavian or femoral veins.

These devices are used for long-term venous access for continuous and intermittent fluids and where peripheral vascular access is problematic.

Withdrawing blood from a central line

Although you can withdraw blood from a central line, this process is often only conducted when no alternative exists and through a dedicated lumen – that is, a lumen not used for drug administration or for any other purpose. Withdrawing blood from a central line is conducted under a strict aseptic technique.

Each hospital has its own policy, but here's the general technique:

1. **Place the patient in the supine position on the bed.**
2. **Use an aseptic technique throughout the procedure.**
3. **Clean the access port/hub with cleaning fluid, such as 2% chlorhexidine with 70% isopropyl alcohol or iodine.**
4. **Aspirate 6–10 ml of blood from the device from adults (less in children depending on their age/size) and discard.**
5. **Take the blood samples (depending on age/size).**
6. **Flush the device with 0.9% sodium chloride using the push-pause technique (see the earlier section 'Making the job easier') and maintain positive pressure in the catheter.**
7. **Replace with a sterile bung.**
8. **Document your actions.**

Caring for a central line

You must maintain patency for all central lines, using fluids such as 0.9% sodium chloride or heparinised saline. Short-term CVADs should be flushed every 12 hours, Long-term catheters and more temporary CVADs (used in treatments such as haemodialysis, continuous renal replacement therapies, plasmapheresis and the removal and return of blood plasma from the circulation) can be flushed weekly, unless occlusion problems exist or manufacturer's guidance states otherwise. After blood withdrawal, administer 10–20 millilitres of the flushing solution using a push-pause motion to create turbulence, to remove debris from the internal catheter.

You need to perform this procedure using a positive pressure technique, achieved by maintaining pressure on the plunger of the syringe and at the same time disconnecting the syringe from the injection site. This approach prevents reflux of blood into the tip of the device, reducing the risk of clot occlusion.

Secure the central line well (often with a stabilisation device) to prevent movement and cover with a sterile dressing (often transparent or lint-free gauze): inspect the site regularly. Document all care in the central line care plan and/or notes.

Observe for any signs of complications, such as the following:

- ✔ Change in heart rate or regularity
- ✔ Change of respiratory rate
- ✔ Pain – localised or referred
- ✔ *Pyrexia* (high temperature)
- ✔ Swelling
- ✔ Tingling in fingers, shooting pain down arm or paralysis

Removing a central line

You usually remove the central line with the patient laying on his back with a pillow under the back. In some cases you conduct the removal as follows:

- ✔ **Trendelenburg position:** The patient lays flat on his back with the head lower than the pelvis.
- ✔ **Valsalva manoeuvre:** The patient exhales forcibly while keeping the mouth and nose closed. The Valsalva manoeuvre raises the inter-thoracic pressure, which helps to prevent an air embolus occurring during the removal of the catheter. You then apply pressure to the site to help stop the bleeding.

Chapter 17

Administering Blood Components

. . . .

. . . .

*N*ot many people's feelings about blood are neutral. On the one hand, plenty hate it and a few even pass out at the sight of a drop (I hope not many nurses though!). On the other hand, a few just lurve it. Yes, beware of vampires, because this chapter's all about blood!

I introduce you to the blood types and the national requirements. I also walk you through the blood collecting and administering procedures.

When administering packed red blood cells, plasma or fresh frozen plasma, this clinical skill comes under the intravenous umbrella, albeit with its own set of National Guidelines.

Introducing Blood Types

When receiving blood products, patients are essentially receiving a tissue transplant, due to the fact that blood is classed as a tissue part. Therefore, if this tissue doesn't match the recipient, the patient's body rejects the product with fatal consequences.

You can see why knowing your blood groups is so important. Here are the main ones:

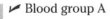

✔ Blood group A

✔ Blood group B

  ✔ Blood group AB

  ✔ Blood group O

Some rarer blood groups are also floating about, such as the following:

  ✔ Blood group C

  ✔ Blood group E

  ✔ Blood group FY

  ✔ Blood group JK

  ✔ Blood group K

  ✔ Blood group S

The antibody known as the *D Rhesus antigen* (*Rh D* to its friends) is also crucial in blood groups. If this antigen sticks to one of the blood groups, the blood group is known as *positive*. If the antigen is absent, the blood group is *negative*.

Blood group O is the most popular guy in the gang because almost half (48 per cent) of the UK population have this blood group: O negative blood group is known as *the universal donor* because you can give it to people with all the other blood groups without causing harm (in most cases).

But if you give B group blood to somebody who's O blood group, the person will die.

Table 17-1 shows the blood-group compatibility of red blood cells for the main blood groups. For example, recipients with blood group A can receive blood donated from individuals with blood groups A and O.

Table 17-1	Blood Group Compatibility for Recipients (Down the Left-Hand Side) and Donors (Along the Top)			
Blood Group	*A*	*B*	*AB*	*O*
A	Yes	No	No	Yes
B	No	Yes	No	Yes
AB	Yes	Yes	Yes	Yes
O	No	No	No	Yes

Being on Top of Blood Transfusion Requirements

Strict regulation is in place within the UK concerning blood matters: from the Department of Health (DOH), the National Patient Safety Agency (NPSA) as well as European Directives. The NPSA are the legislators that oversee the Blood Transfusion practice.

Here are the precise Acts comprising the national requirements:

- ✔ **Department of Health:** Better Blood Transfusion III (2007)
- ✔ **NPSA:** Right Blood, Right Patient (2006)
- ✔ **EC Directive:** 2002/98/EC (Blood Service Quality Reassurance 2005)

The Serious Hazards of Transfusion (SHOT) organisation also oversees the practice of blood transfusion. It collects data from across the UK on all reported transfusion reactions, adverse events or *near-miss* events (when something almost went wrong during the blood transfusion procedure).

Being aware of near-miss events means that everyone can learn from them – and not repeat the same mistakes.

Satisfying the national requirements for blood transfusion

The national requirements state that anyone taking part in the blood transfusion process must have received training in blood transfusion and been competency-assessed in one or all of the assessments, which come under the four main categories in Table 17-2. This applies to people only collecting the blood (for example, a healthcare assistant or porter; see the later section 'Following the required collection procedure') and those administering it to a patient (for example, a midwife or nurse).

These national requirements state that staff must undertake their blood transfusion training every two years and be competency-assessed every two years. Lead Practitioners, who are responsible for assessing their colleagues in their clinical areas, need to attend this training annually.

Table 17-2	Blood Transfusion Competency Assessments		
Competency	*Tick Box If Competency Required*	*Date Competency Completed*	*Review Date = 2 Years Time*
Obtaining a venous blood sample			
Organising receipt of blood products			
Collection of blood products			
Preparation and administration			

Individuals need to have read policies and protocols related to the blood transfusion process and how to report incidents. They also require an understanding of the appropriate use of blood products, the alternatives available and consent issues. Plus, staff should have information and knowledge around local, regional and national audits.

Further aspects of the requirements relate to the fact that areas have to keep records for 30 years and detail issues concerning storage, transportation and traceability of blood products.

Strict protocols also apply to the amount of blood a surgeon can use during the surgery (non-emergency situations). For example, for surgeons undertaking an elective renal transplant, only one unit of packed red blood cells (PRBC) is to be used, if the patient's haemoglobin (Hb) is under 8. Neurosurgeons can only put two units aside during a craniotomy procedure for trauma and an orthopaedic surgeon can only have two units of red blood cells for a hip replacement. No universal PRBC bag size exists: they're variable and for an adult can be from 200 to 575 millilitres – hence health professionals refer to a bag as a unit.

Emergency situations are a different kettle of fish, because more blood may be needed to preserve life.

Obtaining consent

A patient must agree to a transfusion and have signed a consent form (unless in extreme circumstances, such as life-or-death situations). Usually the doctor obtains this consent, but specialised nurses who've undertaken specific training and been approved to do so, can as well.

The person obtaining the consent from the patient must explain, as part of this consent procedure, the indication for the transfusion: in other words, why the patient requires it and the risks, benefits and alternatives.

Obtaining valid consent involves knowing that the following criteria have been met:

- ✔ Does the patient have enough information to make the decision?
- ✔ Does the patient have enough capacity to make the decision?
- ✔ Has the patient made a free choice?

If these three tests haven't been met, valid consent hasn't been given. Of course, certain 'best interests' factors can come into play, where the medical staff state that the patient requires the care being offered and without it can die (as well as issues around 'mental capacity'), but I'd need two more chapters to cover all that! If you do want further information along these lines, you can find it at www.legislation.go.uk.

To help you explain the blood transfusion process accurately so that patients can give valid consent, see the diagrammatic representation of the stages in Figure 17-1.

Patients should also be given any appropriate information leaflets – many are available in a variety of languages. Here's just a selection:

- ✔ 'Will I need a blood transfusion?'
- ✔ 'Information for patients needing irradiated blood'
- ✔ 'Information for patients receiving an unexpected blood transfusion'
- ✔ 'A Parent's Guide – Children receiving a blood transfusion'
- ✔ 'Will my baby need a blood transfusion?'
- ✔ 'Will your child need a plasma transfusion?'
- ✔ 'Blood Groups and Red Cell Antibodies in Pregnancy'

Tracing the Blood Transfusion Procedures

Doctors or appropriately trained specialised nurses and midwives make blood transfusion requests for the specific required blood.

All blood received from a donor is filtered and cleaned, but certain patients need this process to be more vigilant, due to immunosuppressive medical conditions, such as receiving chemotherapy:

- ✔ **Irradiated blood:** Administered to babies in-utero and for individuals requiring a blood transfusion with Hodgkinson's disease and other immunosuppressive conditions.

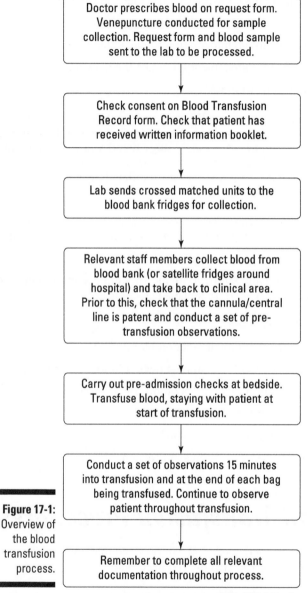

Figure 17-1:
Overview of
the blood
transfusion
process.

✔ **Cytomegalovirus (CMV) blood:** A type of herpes simplex virus, related
to the common cold sore. Most individuals have this virus in their
system and it causes no harm to those with a strong immune system.
But to those with a weakened immune system, this virus in the blood

can cause harm, and so it needs to undergo extra processes to remove the virus in the donor blood.

✔ **Washed cells blood:** Where the plasma proteins are washed away from the plasma, leaving the cells only. This process is performed for patients requiring a transfusion who've had a reaction to a previous transfusion, where something in the donor plasma caused a reaction to the recipient. This process is expensive to undertake and is performed by the National Blood Service.

Performing the sample collection

After a request for a blood transfusion or blood product has been made, a sample of the patient's blood is obtained: in other words, venepuncture (see Chapter 11). This sample is required to *cross match* the blood so that the patient receives the correct blood group donation.

Usually only one sample is required but if the patient has never received a blood product previously, two samples are taken, with two separate request forms. These blood samples can be collected five minutes apart or a day or two later.

The blood for the cross match must be collected into the appropriate blood bottle (as I describe in Chapter 11). For a sample collection, usually 6 millilitres is sent to the laboratory, or 2.7 millilitres for paediatrics and 1 millilitre for neonates.

Staff must be trained in venepuncture to collect this sample and have been assessed as competent. They should also renew their venepuncture skills frequently, as in all their clinical skills, to remain competent.

When the blood is ready for collection, the member of staff organising the receipt of the blood/blood product must undertake key tasks before the blood is collected, including the following:

✔ Checking the consent documentation

✔ Documenting baseline observations on the patient

✔ Ensuring that venous access has been obtained and that this cannula/central line is *patent* (not blocked and ready to receive the transfusion)

The member of staff then asks the patient to state her full name and date of birth and checks that all the information on the identity band and hospital documentation and blood transfusion form is correct, and that this document is fully completed. In this case, check the patient's notes/care plans and with colleague/s and the patient that this is the correct person.

Take extra care with patients who're unable to respond, may be unconscious or have any communication difficulties: *two* competent members of staff must check the identity band, hospital documentation and blood transfusion form.

Before sending a member of staff to collect blood from the blood fridge or a blood product from the laboratory, the doctor, registered nurse, midwife or operating department practitioner (ODP) needs to ensure that the person being sent has undertaken the appropriate training and been assessed as competent for the task.

Following the required collection procedure

The following appropriately trained and competent individuals can be asked to collect red blood cells – after training and competency assessment, and depending on hospital policies and procedures (in some hospitals only porters can collect blood):

- ✔ Assistant practitioner (AP) and trainee AP
- ✔ Healthcare assistant
- ✔ Operating department practitioner (ODP) and student ODP
- ✔ Perioperative ancillary workers
- ✔ Registered or student nurses/midwife
- ✔ Ward clerk/receptionist

Blood components can also be collected by general porters in many hospital trusts, such as Fresh Frozen Plasma (FFP) and platelets.

Some hospitals have the blood collected direct from the blood bank, whereas other larger hospitals may have satellite fridges around the hospital.

When going to the fridge or lab to collect red blood cells for transfusion, the blood transfusion record document must be checked with the blood bank register for the patient's identification: first name, surname, hospital number and date of birth. Any discrepancies must be reported immediately to the blood bank.

The blood bank register informs the collector where in the fridge the blood can be located, for example, 'on the third shelf'. As soon as the blood has been removed, close the fridge door immediately in order to keep the fridge within the cold chain, meaning keeping the temperature between 2–6 degrees Celsius.

If more than one unit of blood has been prepared for the patient, remove the unit at the front first, but only take one unit at a time for general ward use. Theatre porters can remove all the units prepared for the patient, transporting this amount in a specialised cooling bag to maintain the cold-chain temperature.

The unit at the front should have a Compatibility Report form attached, which is to be taken back to the ward area. The collector signs the blood bank register, stating that the bag of blood has been removed and by whom. The blood should be popped into a transport bag to take back to the clinical area.

The collector needs to check the blood, looking for any leaks, discolouration or clots. She also needs to check the expiry date. If the expiry date on the bag is today's date, the blood can still be administered as long as it's transfused before midnight. All units of blood generally need to be administered over three to four hours (preferably three).

The collector takes the blood back to the clinical area and gives it to the person who requested the blood collection. The Blood Transfusion Record sheet must then be completed, stating that the blood has been received.

Don't leave the bag of blood unattended. After the blood has been removed from the fridge, this bag must start to be administered within 30 minutes. If the blood is no longer required, it must be taken back to the blood fridge/lab and signed back in the blood bank register.

Ensuring that the administration procedure is correct

The blood is checked (usually by two members of appropriate staff, but in some areas only one person) so that the ward-ID, the lab register and details on the blood bag match; after which, the blood can be administered.

People who can undertake these checks include doctors, registered nurses, registered midwifes and operating department practitioners. In many clinical areas assistant practitioners can only second check and not administer the blood. Students can check as a third person, but not sign any of the documentation. This is all dependent on individual hospital policies and procedures. Infection control procedures must be adhered to at all times.

When preparing for the transfusion, the staff member must check the patient's identification again, asking her to give her full name and date of birth. The hospital number should also be checked, as well as the Blood

Transfusion Record, details on the blood unit, compatibility label and Compatibility Report form, and the product integrity and special requirements (if requested).

If a CMV negative bag was requested, the bag of blood has the wording 'CMV Neg' on the front label. All the bar codes on the blood unit are to enable a full audit trial – vein-to-vein traceability – using a pulse tracking system.

Observing the monitoring procedure

When the transfusion has started, the Compatibility Report form is completed, stating who administered the transfusion, who undertook all the bedside checks and the date and time that the transfusion was started. After the bag of blood has been transfused, the date and time the transfusion finished is also recorded on this form.

On the unit of blood collected from the fridge, a 'traceability' label is attached, which contains a peel-off sticker section to be placed on the register document. This form usually gets photocopied with the original sheet being sent to the Blood Transfusion centre in order for these records to be kept for 30 years.

Even if the patient received just one drop from the blood unit, this document must be completed.

Drugs must never be added to blood bags under any circumstances, because it can cause damage to the cells or cause the blood/blood product to clot. Also, if the patient has a reaction – how can you tell whether the blood or the drug is causing the problem?

The patient has a second set of observations performed after 15 minutes of the start of the transfusion and a third set of observations performed at the end of transfusion. The observation chart should state '15 min transfusion' and 'End of transfusion'. The pre-transfusion set of observations (the first set) should also have 'pre-transfusion' written onto the observation chart. If a patient is unconscious, more frequent observations should be performed.

Routine transfusions need to be given between the daylight hours of 8 a.m. and 8 p.m. A *volumetric pump* is used to transfuse the blood, with blood warmers employed for children and anyone with cold antibodies: for example, hypothermic patients.

Use sterile blood IV administration sets to administer PRBC, because they contain filters (unlike 'clear' fluid IV administration sets). The set is changed within 12 hours to prevent bacterial growth. Most trust policies require platelet administration sets to be changed after every unit.

Retain all empty blood bags for 24 hours subsequent to the transfusion in case the patient experiences an adverse reaction. In this event, the lab requires the bag back for testing. If platelets are to be transfused, a specialised administration set is recommended (see Table 17-3), where the 'dead space' is less (affording less waste of product).

Table 17-3	Blood and Blood Product Administration Set Information	
Component	**Filter Size**	**Comment**
Packed Red Cells and Autologous Red Cells	170–200-micron filter (blood administration set)	Autologous is blood collected from patient and re-transfused back to same patient.
Platelets	170–200-micron filter (blood administration set); specialist platelet administration sets are available and recommended.	Labs often supply platelet administration sets with the platelets; usually transfused over 30–60 minutes per bag.
Fresh Frozen Plasma (FFP)	170–200-micron filter (blood administration set)	Thawed in lab by blood bank staff.
Granulocytes	170–200-micron filter (blood administration set)	Type of small white blood cells with small protein granules present.
Cryoprecipitate	170–200-micron filter (blood administration set) or platelet administration set	Platelet administration set has a much smaller priming volume and is suitable for cryoprecipitate. This is FFP that has been thawed and obtained by collecting the precipitate when centrifuged.
Human Albumin Solution (HAS)	Usually a standard 'clear fluid' administration-giving set	Albumin transports hormones, fatty acids and other compounds, buffers pH and maintains osmotic pressure within the body. HAS constitutes about half of the blood serum protein.
IV immunoglobulin	15-micron filter vented administration set supplied by drug manufacturer.	Given to immune-deficient patients to maintain adequate antibody levels to prevent infection. Used to treat a number of medical conditions.

Storage of blood products

Here's storage information for red blood cells, platelets and FFP (Fresh Frozen peas, sorry, I mean Plasma – I must be hungry!):

- **Red blood cells:** Kept for 35 days and stored at 2–6 degrees Celsius. All transfusion needs to be transfused within four hours and can only be used 30 minutes after being removed from the fridge and started on the patient.

- **Platelets:** Kept at room temperature and gently agitated so that the cells don't start to stick together. They're stored at 20–24 degrees Celsius for up to seven days. This transfusion is started immediately as soon as it has been obtained and is usually transfused over 30–60 minutes per bag.

- **Fresh Frozen Plasma (FFP):** Stored at minus 30 degrees Celsius for up to three years and thawed by the blood bank staff. This transfusion needs to be started immediately and completed within four hours of collection.

Dealing with adverse effects

Tell transfusion patients to report to staff any side effects, such as shivering, itching, rash, flushing, shortness of breath or generally feeling unwell; all these signs can indicate a possible adverse reaction to the transfusion. The staff member should stay with the patient, observing as the first few millilitres of blood go through, because this is when the patient may first show signs of side effects.

If an adverse reaction is being experienced, stop the transfusion immediately and contact a doctor. One of first indicators of a reaction is a temperature rise of 1 degree Celsius. Check the patient's compatibility label and ID band, reassess the unit for contamination and perform a full set of observations. Also, record the adverse reaction in the patient's notes. Complete all appropriate documentation and inform the blood bank, returning the transfused unit if the doctor requests you to do so.

The doctor may prescribe anti-histamines and paracetamol and request that the transfusion can commence, at a slower rate. Primarily the patient needs to be offered reassurance.

Chapter 18

Reducing Infections and Needle Injuries

In This Chapter

▶ Looking at infection control issues

▶ Avoiding sharps injuries

*I*ntravenous (IV) therapy is regarded as a high-risk area of clinical practice due to the complication of infection, specifically the risk of causing direct microbial entry into the bloodstream. The result can be life-threatening complications such as bacteraemias/septicaemia.

Practitioners involved in IV therapy have to understand that the majority of these infections are avoidable, as long as they adhere to good practice throughout the IV process.

This chapter looks at infection control issues and principles that minimise the risks of infection. I also cover health and safety when using *sharps* (injection needles and the like), which can cause serious injury.

Keeping the Bugs at Bay

Know your enemy! Micro-organisms include bacteria and viruses:

- **Bacteria:** Can be broken down into two major categories:
  - Good bacteria, which live on skin and in the digestive tract
  - Bad bacteria, for example, Legionnaire's disease, pimples and boils
- **Viruses:** Smaller organisms including norovirus, also known as 'winter vomiting viruses' and 'Norwalk'.

Good bacteria can turn bad if they migrate to parts of the body they should never be (like a grade-A student lured into a seedy nightclub!).

In this section you get as close as you'd ever want to micro-organisms, as I discuss all sorts of infections including sepsis and phlebitis, and infection risks.

Meeting micro-organisms

Patients can suffer from bacterial infection due to the following two organisms:

- ✔ **Endogenous organisms:** Already present on the person's body.
- ✔ **Exogenous organisms:** Developed or originated outside the body.

The majority of healthcare associated infections (HCAIs) are endogenous in origin; for example, *staphylococcus epidermidis* (normal flora on the skin) entering the bloodstream after catching a ride on a peripheral cannula due to someone not cleaning the skin correctly prior to insertion.

The consequences of patients acquiring HCAIs are as follows:

- ✔ **Longer in-patient stays:** Owing to patients needing treatment for the infection and/or being too poorly to be discharged.
- ✔ **Increased financial costs:** To the patient and the NHS.
- ✔ **Negative patient experience:** 'I only came in for a minor op and now I feel so unwell!'
- ✔ **Increased morbidity and mortality rates:** Infection can have a devastating effect on immuno-compromised patients.

Table 18-1 shows some infectious micro-organisms associated with IV therapy.

Table 18-1	Micro-organisms Associated with IV Therapy
Micro-organism	*Information*
Methicillin-resistant staphylococcus aureus (MRSA)	Type of bacteria commonly found on skin and/or in the noses of healthy people: if healthy, colonisation doesn't cause problems. When MRSA enters the body (for example, through breaks in the skin), it can cause delayed wound healing. If it enters lungs, it can cause pneumonia. Unfortunately, most strains of staphylococcus aureus are now resistant to penicillin. Creams, shampoos and mouth antibiotics (nystatin) are used to get rid of the infection. AB (antibiotics) = vancomycin and teicoplanin (via IV).

Micro-organism	Information
Escherichia coli (E. coli)	Friendly bacteria, providing body with many vitamins, such as Vitamin K. However, Strain 0157 is potentially fatal. The bacteria live in the lower intestines of mammals (gut flora) such as humans and cattle, and are passed on by eating infected food and liquid. This risk can be minimised by good food-handling practices, cooking meat properly, and keeping raw and cooked meats apart.
Pseudomonas	A genus of gram-negative aerobic bacteria. Pseudomonas aeruginosa is found in burn wounds and urinary tract infections and accumulations of pus.
Enterococcus	A genus of gram-positive anaerobic bacteria of the family previously classified as streptococcus. Found in urinary tract infections and infective endocarditis.

Avoiding infections associated with IV drug administration

When administering IV therapy to your patients, you're opening up a port of entry for the micro-organisms to enter through the access device, increasing the risk of developing an infection. Factors influencing the increased risk of developing an infection include the following:

- ✔ Inadequate hand hygiene

- ✔ Multiple cannulation insertions

- ✔ *Re-palpation* (touching the skin again and contaminating it after cleaning the skin) of proposed site immediately before insertion

- ✔ Length of time the cannula is in-situ

- ✔ Type of cannula (due to longer-term devices presenting higher risk factors) peripheral, central, Hickman

- ✔ Contamination of injection ports and *bungs* ('stoppers' at the end of devices used to inject medication through)

Watching those hands

Hand hygiene is the single most important infection control measure that healthcare workers can carry out to reduce *hospital-acquired infections* (HAIs, the infections people 'acquire' in hospital). You have to perform this activity correctly, using the six-point hand-wash technique I describe here.

Liquid soap is regarded as the gold standard in hand washing, because bars of soap, in a communal place, contain skin cells and so on from the previous user and are therefore an infectious risk in themselves. Yuk!

Here I take you through the six-point hand-wash technique:

1. **Wet your hands under a running tap and then add liquid soap: rub hands together, palm to palm, to create lather.**

2. **Rub the back of each hand with the palm of the other hand with your fingers interlaced.**

3. **Rub the tips of your fingers in the opposite palm in a circular motion.**

4. **Rub each thumb clasped in the opposite hand, using a rotational movement.**

5. **Rub each wrist with the opposite hand.**

6. **Rinse thoroughly with water under running tap and then dry your hands well with paper towels.**

This technique takes only a matter of seconds to perform, but every part of your working tools – the hands – have been cleaned! Use this same six-point hand washing technique for applying alcohol gel.

Wet your hands first. You need to wash off, and slough off, as much as you can – including contaminants and dead skin cells. If you don't perform this process effectively, you may as well not do it at all. MRSA sits on your skin cells for up to three hours: you have to wash your hands vigorously to remove all the bugs.

Getting 'naked to the elbow'

Conduct a 'naked to the elbow' approach when washing hands. (I don't mean naked from the toes up to the elbow! That would be a step too far!) *Naked to the elbow* means that everything below the elbow to the tips of the fingers has to be clear of watches, rings (apart from plain wedding bands, which are permitted for cultural reasons), nail varnish and anything else, because all such items can be a infection risk, carrying germs.

You need to conduct hand washing regularly through the day, even if you haven't been involved in any clinical task. The World Health Organisation devised the '5 Moments for Hand Hygiene', which defines the key moments when healthcare workers should carry out hand hygiene:

✔ Before touching a patient

✔ Before clean/aseptic procedures are to be used

✔ After body fluid exposure/risk

✔ After touching a patient

✔ After touching a person's surroundings

Considering the chain of infection

Infections occur when six elements are present in sequential order, often referred to as the *chain of infection*.

Breaking the chain

Breaking any one of the links to the following six-link chain prevents the spread of infection:

1. **Causative agents:** Any micro-organism capable of producing disease – includes bacteria, viruses, fungi and parasites.

2. **Reservoir:** Supports the causation chink in the chain, allowing micro-organisms to survive and multiply. Infectious reservoirs are plentiful in the healthcare setting and include patients, staff, visitors, medical equipment, the environment, vascular access devices (peripheral cannulae, central venous catheters), IV solutions and drugs. The reservoir also includes food and water.

3. **Portal of exit from reservoir (means of exit):** Allows the infectious agent to leave the reservoir. The portal of exit is usually the site where the micro-organism grows, for example, the blood and other body fluids, such as faeces and urine, secretions and skin scales from the patient's skin.

4. **Mode of transmission:** Where the micro-organism moves from the reservoir to a new host. Micro-organisms can be transmitted or acquired in a variety of ways, including direct and indirect contact and contact with air/droplets in the environment. In IV therapy, the main routes of transmission are:

   • Direct contact – hands of the healthcare worker

   • Indirect contact – contaminated equipment, fluids, IV drugs or infusates

   • Puncture of the skin – inoculation/blood borne

5. **Portal of entry into host (means of entry):** The path by which micro-organisms invade a susceptible host – usually the same as the means of exit in step 3. In IV therapy, any intravenous device, such as a peripheral cannula or central venous catheter, creates an additional portal of entry into a patient's body, increasing the chance of infection risk.

6. **Susceptible host:** Anyone at risk of developing an infection. The human body tries to fend off any invading micro-organisms, but certain categories of individuals are at risk if this defence mechanism isn't fully functioning, or variables predispose individuals to an increased risk of infection, including:

- Antimicrobial treatments

- Chronic disease, such as diabetes, liver disease

- Compromised immune system

- Elderly

- Extended length of hospital stay

- Infants

- IV drug users

- Surgery (wound sites)

- Vascular access devices

This chain illustrates why hand hygiene (see the earlier section 'Watching those hands') is the single most important infection control measure to ward off micro-organism contamination. Breaking a link in the chain of infection stops the infection in its tracks and prevents it from spreading. If the infection isn't stopped, it can progress up the infection scale (refer to Figure 18-1).

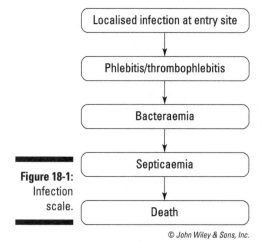

Figure 18-1: Infection scale.

© John Wiley & Sons, Inc.

Decontaminating equipment

Cleaning equipment is another key element in the fight against infection. Choosing the correct process of decontamination is important for this process to be effective:

- ✔ **Cleaning:** Physically removes contamination. Needs to be undertaken before disinfecting/sterilisation.

- ✔ **Disinfection:** Reduces the number of micro-organisms. May not deactivate certain viruses and bacterial spores.

- ✔ **Sterilisation:** Renders an object free from viable micro-organisms, including viruses and bacterial spores.

When wearing personal protection equipment, follow these key principles:

- ✔ You can use alcohol gel, if no water is available, until you're able to wash hands with soap and water.

  Never use gels more than three times without then washing your hands with soap and water. Also, don't use alcohol gels for outbreaks of C. difficile, diarrhoea/vomiting and/or MRSA: use only soap and water.

- ✔ Aprons are single use – don't wear more than once.

- ✔ Wear clean apron for each task.

- ✔ Remove appropriately and reapply appropriately.

- ✔ Use the appropriate gloves for the task – for example, nitrile (latex free), vinyl.

Infecting the blood or body: Sepsis

Sepsis is a bacterial infection in the bloodstream or body tissues, usually after a localised infection or injury. The most common sites of infection leading to sepsis are the lungs, urinary tract, abdomen and pelvis. Sepsis can occur after surgery, after an IV drip has been inserted or a central line, or during or following urinary catheter insertion.

The 'Sepsis 6' initiative is part of a government campaign to lower the mortality rate of sepsis in all patients. Each year in the UK around 37,000 people die as a result of the condition.

Symptoms

The symptoms of sepsis usually develop quickly and can include the following, which may occur simultaneously:

- Chills and shivers
- Elevated temperature
- Fast breathing rate
- Tachycardia

If not treated quickly enough, symptoms can progress to septic shock and blood pressure dropping to dangerously low levels. The following symptoms can develop within hours:

- Change in mental state, such as confusion or disorientation
- Cold, clammy and pale mottled skin
- Decreased urine production
- Diarrhoea
- Feeling dizzy or faint
- Loss of consciousness
- Nausea and vomiting
- Severe breathlessness
- Severe muscle pain
- Slurred speech

Assessment

The patient requires a full assessment, using the National Early Warning Score (NEWS) observation tool (flip to Chapter 7 for details). Check to see whether any two or more of the following are present with a NEWS of greater than 3 or a clinical suspicion of infection:

- Temperature less than 36 degrees Celsius or more than 38 degrees Celsius
- Respiratory rate more than 20 breaths per minute
- Acutely altered mental state
- Heart rate more than 90 bpm

If YES to two or more of these being present – measure lactate (by venepuncture).

Then if results then show:

- ✔ Systolic BP less than 90
- ✔ Mean arterial pressure less than 65
- ✔ Lactate greater than 2
- ✔ INR greater than 1.5
- ✔ Urine output less than 0.5 ml/kg/hr
- ✔ Or other evidence of organ dysfunction

Analysis of results

If NO to these results, sepsis is identified and treatment would begin and patient monitored closely.

If YES to these results, the indication is severe sepsis with a 35 per cent mortality rate. Treatment is to initiate the Sepsis 6.

Treatment = Sepsis 6

Severe sepsis and septic shock are medical emergencies. The government initiative is called 'Sepsis 6', because of the six-step treatment of severe sepsis:

1. **Give 15 litres of oxygen via facemask with reservoir – unless oxygen restrictions apply.**

   During sepsis your body's demand for oxygen goes up.

2. **Give IV fluids, 500–1,000 millilitres bolus of Hartman's; larger bolus if systolic blood pressure is less than 90 or lactate greater than 4.**

   During sepsis, your body requires increased amounts of fluids to prevent dehydration and kidney failure.

3. **Take blood cultures, but follow hospital guidelines; culture other sites as clinically indicated, for example, sputum, wound, swabs and so on.**

   Blood culture testing is used to identify the bacteria present to then guide the treatment.

4. **Treat with IV antibiotics, but follow hospital guidelines – delay in administration increases mortality.**

   IV antibiotic administration is the main treatment for sepsis and should be started within the first hour of diagnosis.

5. **Take lactate and bloods: lactate on arterial or venous samples, full blood count, Us and Es (urea and electrolyte blood test used to screen for kidney failure and dehydration), liver function tests, clotting screen (INR and APTT blood clotting tests).**

   You may want to flip to Chapter 11 to read on these blood tests and glucose.

6. **Monitor urine output measurements using fluid charts.**

   Knowing how much urine the kidneys are producing is important to assess for signs of kidney failure. This may mean urine catheterisation – putting a tube into the bladder. Take mid-stream urine sample or catheter sample and perform an urinalysis (using test strips).

Performing a visual inspection of phlebitis

Phlebitis is the inflammation of the vein, causing pain and swelling due to the trauma. Superficial phlebitis is most often caused during cannula insertion due to IV therapy.

Phlebitis comes in three categories:

- ✔ **Bacterial phlebitis:** Inflammation of a vein caused by bacterial infection during cannula insertion or after the procedure.

- ✔ **Chemical phlebitis:** Irritation instigated by drug therapy with the vein/cannula being too small for the volume or type of solution.

- ✔ **Mechanical phlebitis:** Caused by the irritation of the cannula in the vein (often the cannula is too large and not secured correctly).

When a patient has an access device in-situ allowing for IV therapy to be instigated, checking the access site regularly is important. Peripherally inserted cannulae use the assessment tool known as the 'Infusion phlebitis score assessment'. This tool, known as the Visual Infusion Phlebitis (VIP) score, observes the access device insertion site and arm/hand for any signs of infection. The assessment documentation generally consists of the observed signs and actions in Table 18-2. This system was developed by Andrew Jackson (not the seventh President of the USA, but a consultant nurse in 1998).

Table 18-2		Visual Infusion Phlebitis Score
Signs	**Score**	**Actions**
IV site appears healthy	0	No sign of phlebitis; continue to observe cannula
Slight pain near IV site or slight redness (erythema) near IV site	1	Possibly first sign of phlebitis; continue to observe cannula
Observing two of the following: Pain near IV site; erythema; swelling	2	Early stage of phlebitis; re-site cannula
Pain along path of cannula; erythema and induration (hardening of soft tissue)	3	Medium stage of phlebitis; re-site cannula; consider treatment
All the following are evident and extensive: Pain along path of cannula; erythema; induration; palpable venous cord	4	Advanced stage of phlebitis; thrombophlebitis; re-site cannula; consider treatment
All the following are evident and extensive: Pain along path of cannula; erythema; induration; palpable venous cord; pyrexia (high temperature)	5	Advanced stage of thrombophlebitis; initiate treatment; re-site cannula

If a patient complains of pain when flushing the cannula, remember these important principles:

✔ Don't ignore a painful cannula site.

✔ Pain can be associated with phlebitis.

✔ Pain can be associated with poor location, for example, over a joint.

✔ Site doesn't have to look painful to be painful.

✔ Pain may be drug-induced – for example, wrong dilution or vein irritant.

Staying Sharp to Stay Safe

When handling injection needles, inserting cannula stylets and so on, you need to take great care – not only with the body fluids, but also with the management of these sharps. Injuries caused by needles and other 'sharps' are one of the most common risks to healthcare workers, with 40,000 incidents reported each year.

Minimising and treating needle-stick injuries

A *needle-stick injury* is when the equipment you're using penetrates the skin accidently and causes an injury. The 'sharps' include needles used for injections, scalpels and scissors – in short, medical instruments used day-to-day in healthcare. Sharps contaminated with an injected patients' blood can transmit more than 20 different diseases, such as hepatitis B, C and human immune deficient virus (HIV).

These injuries are often caused by re-sheathing needles, which can be avoided by using the one-handed scoop technique in an injection tray (see Figure 18-2). Used needles should never be re-sheathed.

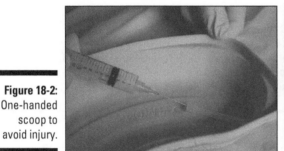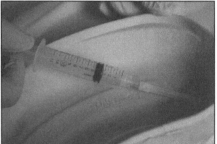

Figure 18-2: One-handed scoop to avoid injury.

© *John Wiley & Sons, Inc.*

Here are a few other tips for avoiding needle-stick injuries:

- ✔ Don't overfill sharps bins.
- ✔ Be extra vigilant when handling sharps to avoid injury.
- ✔ Don't use *pulp trays* (mode of cardboard-type material) but only rigid injection trays.
- ✔ Read the sharps handling policy in your area and know what to do if you're injured.

If you do sustain a needle stick injury, you can follow these steps (but remember your own employer's policy and procedures, too):

1. **Apply first aid.**
2. **Encourage the wound to bleed by squeezing.**
3. **Wash thoroughly with running water.**

4. **Cover the wound with waterproof dressing.**

5. **Contact the help line in your place of work and occupational health can then offer advice.**

6. **Inform your manager and fill out an accident/incident form.**

Disposing of sharps properly

Sharps bins come in all different sharps and sizes (although they're often made of yellow plastic, are permanently sealable when full and have instructions and warnings printed on them). As a user, you need to decide which one is fit for purpose in each situation.

The sharps-bin protocol is as follows:

✔ Assemble sharps bins correctly.

✔ Dispose of sharps at the point of use.

✔ If *you* use it, *you* dispose of it!

✔ Keep sharps bins off the floor and away from public access – especially children!

✔ Never, ever re-sheath used needles.

✔ Only ever fill sharps bins three-quarters full before closing and disposing of them.

✔ Use the temporary closure mechanism when boxes aren't in use and during transport.

✔ Use the trays with integral sharps boxes.

Chapter 19

Checking for IV Therapy Complications

. . . .

In This Chapter

▶ Minimising adverse effects

▶ Managing cannula issues

▶ Maintaining IV safety

. . . .

*P*roblems associated with IV therapy are many and varied. In this chapter I take a look at the complications associated with IV therapy and strategies for management. Specifically I cover potential problems to watch out for when you're administrating medication intravenously, including fluid overload, speed shock, extravasation, infiltration and precipitation.

Avoiding Problems when Administrating IV Medication

This section discusses how you can recognise some of the dangers often associated with IV therapy and how to rectify these problems if they occur.

Of course, the aim at all times is to observe your patients closely so that these issues don't occur in the first place!

Minimising fluid overload (hypervolaemia)

Hypervolaemia (also known as circulatory overload) can occur when too much fluid is being administered to the body or at a higher rate than the body system can absorb or excrete. To assess your patient for hypervolaemia, you need to be vigilant and observe for the following tell-tale signs:

✔ Anxiety

✔ Clamminess

✔ *Cyanosis* (blue or purple colouration) of the lips and nail beds

✔ Distended neck veins

✔ *Dyspnoea* (difficult or laboured breathing), *tachypnoea* (an abnormally rapid breathing rate)

✔ Fluid balance chart shows a wide variance between fluid input and fluid output (a positive balance)

✔ Increased blood pressure recordings/central venous pressure readings

✔ Puffy eyelids and generalised oedema

✔ Respiratory 'rattle sounds' and/or crackles

✔ Weight gain

✔ Wheezing

Management of hypervolaemia includes stopping the IV infusion if still in-situ but leaving the IV access device in place (in case required as part of the management strategy).

Here are some other steps you can take in the case of hypervolaemia:

1. **Contact the medics and require an urgent patient review.**

2. **Communicate the National Early Warning Score (NEWS) to the medical team: it can give a measurable indication of the patient's condition.**

3. **Record the patient's vital signs as frequently as necessary to prevent deterioration in her clinical condition.**

4. **Position the patient in an upright position and give oxygen therapy and consider supplying extra blankets to promote circulation.**

5. **Give the patient continued reassurance.**

6. **Prepare for the medical review team to request patient urinary catheterisation and IV furosemide therapy.**

7. **Document all actions and complete records associated with the patient's adverse effects.**

In Chapter 14, I show you how to recognise the signs and symptoms of hypervolaemia (and hypovolaemia) in general. Chapter 15 looks at how electrolyte disturbances can disrupt normal bodily functioning and the importance of using laboratory testing to assess your patient's fluid and electrolyte status in order to rectify any abnormalities.

Table 19-1 lists some of the most common tests for evaluating fluid status.

Table 19-1	Tests Performed to Evaluate Fluid Status	
Laboratory Test	*Information about the Test*	*Normal Laboratory Value*
Blood serum osmolarity	Measures the balance between water and chemicals dissolved in blood. Determines whether severe dehydration or over-hydration is present.	275–295 mmol*/kg
Haematocrit	Measures the proportion of red blood cells within the blood. Dehydration produces a falsely high haematocrit reading.	42–54% in males; 38–46% in females
Blood urea nitrogen (BUN)	Measures the amount of nitrogen in the blood that comes from the waste product urea. Dehydration can raise BUN levels.	2.1–7.1 mmol/l*
Urine osmolarity	Measures the concentration of particles in urine. Higher levels than normal may indicate dehydration.	Random = 50–1,200 milliosmoles*/kg; 24-hour test = 450–900 milliosmoles*/kg
Urine specific gravity (SG)	Measures the density of urine compared to water, thereby establishing the kidney's ability to concentrate or dilute. A high urine SG indicates dehydration.	1.001–1.030 (normal range); in neonates, normal urine specific gravity is 1003
Urine sodium	Measures the concentration of sodium in the urine. Determines the kidney's ability to conserve or remove sodium from the urine and is therefore an indicator of hydration status.	40–220 mEq/l/day (milliequivalent litres per day), a measurement of concentration: 1mEq/l = 1 mmol/litre

*mmol/l (millimole/litre) is the amount of substance concentration per litre (a millimole is one thousandth of a mole) and milliosmoles is a medical measurement used to measure solutes: as a solute increases, water decreases.

Avoiding speed shock

Speed shock has nothing to do with watching in wonderment at how fast Usain Bolt runs the 100 metres! In the world of IV therapy, speed shock occurs due to the IV medication being administered too quickly.

Signs and symptoms to observe with a patient in cases of speed shock vary according to the drug, but can include the following:

- ✔ Flushed
- ✔ Irregular pulse
- ✔ Loss of consciousness
- ✔ Shock, cardiac arrest
- ✔ Tight chest

Management in cases of speed shock is similar to that for hypervolaemia in the preceding section:

1. **Discontinue the drug administration if observed speed shock occurs during the administration process.**

2. **Contact the medics and require an urgent patient review.**

3. **Communicate the NEWS to the medical team as a measurable indication of the patient's condition.**

4. **Record the patient's vital signs as frequently as necessary to prevent deterioration in her clinical condition.**

5. **Prepare for resuscitation.**

6. **Document all actions and complete records associated with the patient's adverse effects.**

Furosemide is available in a concentration of 20 milligrams in 2 millilitres. A patient is prescribed 10 milligrams IV as a bolus, to be given at a maximum rate of 4 mg/min. First, what volume of furosemide do you administer?

You use the invaluable What you want divided by What you've got times volume formula from Chapter 8:

10 mg/20 mg × 2 ml = 1 ml

Second, over how many minutes should you give the furosemide?

Dose prescribed 10 mg/Rate 4 mg/min = 2.5

Therefore, the correct timing for this patient is 2½ minutes.

This situation arose in reality and, unfortunately, the patient was given the furosemide as a bolus IV injection in a matter of 5 seconds, causing her to experience permanent tinnitus. The speed-shock symptoms occurred because this rate of drug administration was too fast.

Investigating incompatibility issues

The risk of interactions and incompatibilities is greatest in IV therapy, especially with infusions running over several hours, because the drug and infusate are often in contact with each other for a substantial period of time. (This situation may result in precipitation, which I discuss in the later 'Knowing how to avoid precipitation' section.) For example:

- ✔ Some drugs can lose their potency when exposed to ultraviolet and/or fluorescent light, resulting in the patient not receiving the required dose of medication, for example, amphotericin (used for fungal infections). For this reason, such drugs need to be protected from the light by covering with a bag.

- ✔ Some drugs can become toxic when degraded by light, such as sodium nitroprusside into cyanide. (I knew watching all those episodes of Miss Marple would come in handy one day!)

- ✔ Some drugs need to be diluted with the correct pH solution, because otherwise precipitation can occur, meaning that the drug and solution separate. For instance, sodium chloride 0.9% (normal saline) and water for injection have a neutral pH of 7. Glucose 5% is acidic with a usual pH between 4 and 5.

  As a general rule, acidic drugs are given in 'glucose 5%' and alkaline drugs in 'sodium chloride 0.9%'.

Sodium fusidate is supplied with a vial of buffer to reconstitute the dry powder. This solution can then be added to glucose 5% for infusion. If, however, the powder is reconstituted with glucose 5%, the sodium fusidate precipitates due to the acidic pH.

Examining embolisms

An *embolus* is basically anything that travels through the blood vessels until it reaches a vessel that's too small to let it pass, causing a blockage.

Three types of embolism exist:

- ✔ **Air embolism:** Air bubbles entering the cardiovascular system.

- ✔ **Mechanical:** Broken piece of cannula or glass from ampoule or rubber from ampoule.

- ✔ **Thrombus:** Blood clot particles.

Air embolisms

Air embolism is where a bolus of air enters the venous or arterial bloodstream. If large enough it can lodge in the heart, lungs and brain, resulting in brain damage, a stroke or even death.

As little as 10 millilitres of air may be sufficient to cause serious harm to a patient.

Central venous access devices (CVADs) bring with them an increased risk of air embolism, because air may enter the central venous system through the entire site, travelling directly to the right side of the heart and proving fatal. For this reason, positive pressure must be maintained during flushing and locking procedures.

Priming an IV administration set with fluid is important, because these lines can contain 15–20 millilitres of air.

Mechanical embolisms

When a needle punctures the rubber septum on an ampoule, it picks up small bits of the rubber, which can be inadvertently injected into the patient (called the *coring effect*). Glass vials also bring with them the danger of picking up small shards of glass, which again can be injected into the patient.

Here's how to minimise coring when drawing up medication from an ampoule with rubber septums: after cleaning, insert the needle, bevel up, at an angle of 45–60 degrees. Before completely inserting the needle tip into the ampoule, lift the needle to 90 degrees before proceeding.

Thrombus

A *thrombus* is a solid mass of platelets and/or fibrin and other components of blood that form a mass when the clotting mechanism is activated. This type of embolism occurs when a piece of the thrombus breaks free and is carried towards the heart, lungs or brain. The term *thromboembolus* can mean bits of plaque, fat and other materials that may create a plug *(atherosclerotic plaque)*, blocking an artery delivering blood to the tissues causing *ischemia* (tissue death).

A *pulmonary embolism* is the blockage of the lung's pulmonary artery (or one of its branches) usually by a blood clot, and may be associated with CVADs due to the clot formation around the central catheter close to the right ventricle of the heart, resulting in serious complications and even death.

Discussing drug errors

One of the key tasks of any nurse is to administer medications. Unfortunately, everyone can make mistakes. An error in calculating a dose for IV drug administration can have a devastating effect due to its quick mode of action. In short, you can seriously harm your patients – and even kill them. For this reason, nurses and all practitioners involved in the medication process have to undertake a programme of education.

The Nursing and Midwifery Council (the governing body of these professions) states that two practitioners need to be involved in complex calculations and considers best practice to have two practitioners involved in all but the most basic drug calculations.

If you're administering a continuous infusion and notice a drug error, take the following actions:

- ✔ Stop the infusion if it's still running.

- ✔ Report the error to senior staff, including the doctor and pharmacist.

- ✔ Inform the patient of mistake and offer reassurance.

- ✔ Undertake relevant vital sign observations.

- ✔ Document all actions and complete records associated with patient's drug error.

- ✔ Be honest and never try to hide your mistakes: hiding them can cause more harm to patients and, after all, an antidote may be available.

Here I relate a few real-life cases to show how vigilance is required in IV drug administration. One is a minor drug error and the others more serious.

Minor drug error

Concentrated solutions increase the risk of *thrombophlebitis* (vein inflammation).

A preparation of 1.2 grams of co-amoxiclav used 10 millilitres instead of 20 millilitres of water for injection. The drug didn't dissolve completely because insufficient solvent was used. The result was thrombophlebitis and a thrombus (blood clot), necessitating anticoagulant and thrombolytic medication therapy (IV) and prolonged hospital stay.

Severe drug errors

In one case, the whole contents of a vial containing 125,000 units of heparin were prepared as a continuous infusion, resulting in a five times overdose and a life-threatening haemorrhage.

In another instance, a mental health nurse was visiting her patient in the community to administer his antipsychotic medication for his schizophrenia for oral ingestion. Here are the details:

- **Medication:** Clozapine
- **Prescribed:** 300 mg
- **Presented as:** Suspension 50 mg/ml – in bottles of 14 ml

The nurse administered six bottles, giving the patient 4,200 mg/84 ml. The patient died.

If the nurse had used the formula to work out the amount to administer, she'd have seen that she should've given only 6 millilitres (300 milligrams) of the drug: What you want divided by What you've got times Volume

$$300 \text{ mg}/50 \text{ mg} \times 1 \text{ ml} = 6 \text{ ml}$$

Do you see where she made the mistake? The bottles contained 50 mg in 1 ml of solution and the nurse thought that each 14-ml bottle contained this amount. In fact, the bottles contained 14 ml, which equates to 700 mg of the drug per bottle (700 mg × 6 bottles = 4,200 mg).

I hope you also noticed that this drug was to be administered orally and not intravenously, even though the same formula is used for oral liquid medications and for IVs – which can come in liquid form (or need to be reconstituted into liquid form). Such aspects can save a person's life.

Dealing with Cannula Problems

In order to administer IV drugs, you need first an access device – the most common one being a cannula – your port of entry into the vein. A plethora of problems can occur with these devices, some of which I look at here. I discuss occlusion, infiltration and extravasation (which sounds disconcertedly like a trio of pretentious 1970s prog-rock albums).

Tackling cannula occlusion

Occlusions are where a formation of blood collects at the tip of the access device in the vein and obstructs the flow of fluids through the catheter. They're often associated with central venous lines and peripherally inserted cannulae due to *catheter-related thrombosis.*

To prevent this build-up of blood, you need to initiate regular *flushing* – pushing normal saline through the access device. You use the *push-pause* flushing technique – sometimes called the stop-start technique – where you inject a small of amount of fluid into the IV access device, and then stop for a moment before resuming. This technique prevents a blood clot build-up at the cannula tip.

If the cannula is difficult to flush, *never* force the fluid against resistance, because you can dislodge the clot and cause a thrombotic event.

You can prevent catheter-related thrombosis by observing and reacting to the following key warning signs:

- ✓ Cannula is difficult to flush
- ✓ Infusion runs slowly or stops
- ✓ Cannula is painful
- ✓ IV pump continually alarms

Catheter-related embolism can also occur in central lines, due to the following:

- ✓ **Pinch-off syndrome:** Central line is caught between the juncture of the first rib and the clavicle, pinching and obstructing the catheter to the point of rupture.
- ✓ **Manufacturing defect:** Can be defects in the lumen of the line or the device itself, causing a loss of wall integrity and risk of rupture.

Mechanical embolisms (see the earlier section 'Examining embolisms') can also occlude the cannula, such as when the catheter ruptures and bits from it flow into the bloodstream. You can prevent this problem by never using a syringe smaller than recommended for flushing: for example, using a 10-millilitre syringe to flush.

Getting under the skin: Avoiding infiltration

Infiltration occurs when the cannula dislodges from the vein and the infused substance, which is non-vesicant and therefore not capable of causing tissue death, enters the surrounding tissues. (You may also still hear people using the old term for this problem – *tissuing* – because of the infusate going into the tissues.) If the medication being infused is IV fluids, you may observe swelling of the limb around the peripheral cannula site.

Some of the causes of infiltration include inadequately securing the cannula so that it comes out of the vein, excessive manipulation of the line and vein weakness (such as elderly, fragile veins). Note that the patient often expresses pain when flushing the cannula – the rationale for never ignoring a painful cannula. Listen to what the patient tells you. Other signs and symptoms of infiltration include observing for phlebitis and the patient's cool oedematous extremity.

In CVADs, infiltration can be due to the following: catheter leakage, rupture or fracture; the device perforating the vein; incomplete insertion of the needle into an implanted port; or the needle becoming dislodged from an implanted port.

Management for infiltration consists of the following:

1. **Stop the infusion.**

2. **Inform the medical team for review.**

3. **Give the patient analgesia to manage the pain.**

4. **Position the patient's limb to facilitate comfort – elevate the limb.**

5. **Check the dilution of the drugs/fluids administered (for drug errors).**

6. **Check administration instructions – should the drug have been administered as a bolus or intermittent infusion?**

7. **Assess the cannula insertion site and Visual Infusion Phlebitis (VIP) documentation for any signs of problems.**

8. **Document all actions in the care plans/patient's notes.**

Recognising and managing extravasation

Extravasation occurs when a vesicant substance, which is capable of causing tissue death, is administered into the surrounding tissues. In other words, the cause is the same as for infiltration in the preceding section except that the substance destroys the surrounding tissue.

Vesicant substances are fluids such as phenytoin (which has the same pH as bleach), highly acidic or markedly alkaline medications, and chemotherapy drugs. Vesicant substances can cause tissue necrosis and/or sloughing of the skin. DNA-binding vesicants (such as doxorubicin) bind to nucleic acids in the DNA of healthy cells, resulting in cell death, whereas non-DNA binding vesicants (such as vinca alkaloids) have an indirect rather than direct effect on the cells.

This list contains examples of vesicant substances:

- ✔ **Vinca alkaloids:**
  - Vinblastine
  - Vincristine
  - Vindesine
- ✔ **Group A drugs:**
  - Calcium chloride
  - Calcium gluconate
  - Glucose 50%
  - Hypertonic solutions, such as sodium chloride > 0.9%
  - Sodium bicarbonate > 5%
  - Phenytoin
- ✔ **Group B drugs:**
  - Aciclovir
  - Cefotaxime
  - Diazepam
  - Doxorubicin
  - Epirubicin
  - Mannitol
  - Mitomycin C
  - Potassium chloride > 40 mmol/l
  - Potassium phosphate

The person administering the medication must know the group of drug being administered, because drugs from group A and drugs from group B may require different antidotes. Also, if drugs from group A and group B are mixed, drug A may cause more damage than drug B, and so the antidote would be used for drug A rather than drug B. You may want to read this paragraph again!

Vinca alkaloids are a class of anti-cancer drugs originally derived from the Madagascar periwinkle plant!

Watching for extravasation

Patients most at risk of extravasation include infants, young children and elderly patients. Also at risk are unconscious and sedated patients, those with language issues, patients with fragile veins or who're *thrombocytopenic* (they have a decreased level of thrombocytes, commonly known as platelets, present in the blood), as well as people taking anticoagulant and steroidal medications.

Signs and symptoms of extravasation include the following:

✔ Patient complaining of a burning or stinging pain at the injection site

✔ Swelling at the injection site

✔ IV medication being administered at a sluggish rate or the pump continually alarming

✔ Resistance (usually) felt when administering a bolus injection and possible swelling on the peripherally cannulated limb or absence of blood backflow in the central venous line

Without early detection and treatment, the following symptoms may occur:

✔ Skin blistering (a one-to two-week post-extravasation event)

✔ Peeling and sloughing of the skin (a two-week post-extravasation event)

✔ Tissue necrosis (two-to three-week post-extravasation)

✔ Damage to tendons, joints and nerves

✔ Loss of limb, breast and/or functional and sensory impairment of affected area

Many clinical areas, where vesicant medications are administered, keep extravasation kits, enabling immediate treatment.

Managing extravasation

Management includes the following actions:

1. **Stop the infusion (if still running) immediately.**

2. ***Don't* remove the cannula straightaway, because the residual drug may need to be aspirated through the cannula.**

3. **Inform the medical team for review immediately.**

4. **Conduct observations on the NEWS assessment tool.**

5. **Elevate patient's arm for comfort.**

6. ***Don't* use the same limb if patient requires peripheral cannulation again.**

7. **Document all actions in the care plans/patient's notes.**

Treatment for extravasation depends on the vesicant drug, and so you need to obtain immediate advice from the medical team and pharmaceutical support. I set out the general advice, however, in Figure 19-1.

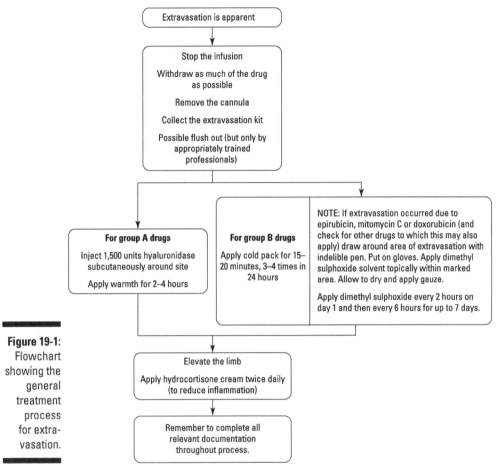

Figure 19-1: Flowchart showing the general treatment process for extravasation.

Extravasation is apparent

Stop the infusion

Withdraw as much of the drug as possible

Remove the cannula

Collect the extravasation kit

Possible flush out (but only by appropriately trained professionals)

For group A drugs

Inject 1,500 units hyaluronidase subcutaneously around site

Apply warmth for 2–4 hours

For group B drugs

Apply cold pack for 15–20 minutes, 3–4 times in 24 hours

NOTE: If extravasation occurred due to epirubicin, mitomycin C or doxorubicin (and check for other drugs to which this may also apply) draw around area of extravasation with indelible pen. Put on gloves. Apply dimethyl sulphoxide solvent topically within marked area. Allow to dry and apply gauze.

Apply dimethyl sulphoxide every 2 hours on day 1 and then every 6 hours for up to 7 days.

Elevate the limb

Apply hydrocortisone cream twice daily (to reduce inflammation)

Remember to complete all relevant documentation throughout process.

Getting Smart with Other IV-Related Precautions

In this section I discuss a couple of general IV issues: avoiding precipitation and managing fluid administration sets correctly.

Knowing how to avoid precipitation

Meteorologically speaking, precipitation is something falling from the sky, such as rain, sleet, snow, hail and drizzle. Get to the point, you're thinking, I don't administer IVs outdoors! Ah, but when you realise that precipitation also means 'falling particles', you can see the relevance to adding drugs to IV bags of fluid.

In this context, *precipitation* is the insufficient mixing of drug and solution in an IV bag. For example, when adding a drug (such as IV amoxicillin) into a bag of IV fluid (such as '0.9% sodium chloride'), you must mix the two substances well to prevent separation. You do so by gently inverting the bag several times, and not by shaking. If performed incorrectly, the patient doesn't receive a consistent dose throughout.

You add potassium chloride to a bag of fluid but fail to mix the contents thoroughly, causing the potassium to fall to the bottom of the bag. The patient receives a whacking great dose of the potassium, causing a potential cardiac arrest.

Figure 19-2 shows the effect of precipitation, where the drug has separated from the fluid.

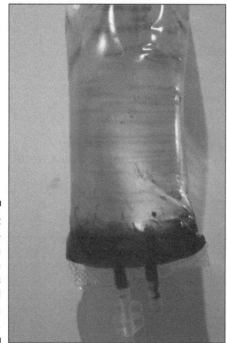

Figure 19-2:
Precipita-
tion – notice
how the
drug has
separated
from the
fluid.

© John Wiley & Sons, Inc.

You may hear people call this effect 'layering', but technically the two terms are slightly different. *Precipitation* is when two IV fluids being mixed together have very different pH values; for example, one is alkaline and one is acidic. *Layering* occurs when two IV fluids with different densities are insufficiently mixed together.

Caring for IV fluid administration sets

To minimise complications when administering IV fluids, observe the following administration line management procedures (though your own healthcare area may have its own protocol):

✔ Ensure that administration sets are appropriate for the administered product.

✔ Check that the administration set is compatible with the infusion pump, if used (staff need to be competent in using the infusion pump devices).

✔ Administration sets need to be dated to alert staff when they require changing. Replace administration sets as follows:

- Crystalloid/maintenance fluid: After 72 hours.

- Total Parenteral Nutrition (TPN): Normally after 24 hours (some 48-hourly bags exist).

- Antibiotics and ward-prepared drug infusions: After 24 hours.

- Blood, blood products and colloid (for example, gelofusine): Immediately following use. Some healthcare areas state blood/platelet administration sets to be changed within 12 hours.

Don't reconnect an administration set after it's disconnected from an access device.

Chapter 20

Meeting Sister Morphine: The Poppy and Pain Management

*F*rom the patients' point of view, pain is simply something they want rid of. For the healthcare professional, however, it can be an important indicator. Pain is often seen as the fifth vital sign and so, as well as assessing patients for their physiological recordings, you need to monitor their pain levels and act on them.

Morphine is the gold standard for all the opiates used in pain control. This chapter looks at administering this highly potent analgesia in its varying forms and routes.

Ouch! Dipping a Toe into a World of Pain

Pain is a multifaceted experience encompassing physical and emotional elements. For this reason, you use pharmacological and non-pharmacological approaches, such as distraction, to reduce patients' experience of pain.

Non-pharmacological methods of managing pain include the following:

✔ Acupuncture

✔ Comfort measures/positioning

✔ Deep breathing exercises

✔ Distraction

Pain pathways and the Pain Gate Theory

To understand pain, you need to know about the *pain pathways*. Hold onto your hat – you may need to read this sidebar more than once.

Pain is first detected by sensory nerve endings (receptors) known as *nociceptors,* which are found throughout the tissues of the body and carry nerve impulses towards the central nervous system (CNS). Picture a car travelling towards the brain. Impulses travel via large myelinated *A-delta* fibres – conducting information at a fast rate – and/or by smaller *C* fibres – conducting information at a slower rate due to their unmyelination. (*Myelin* is a protein and phospholipid material covering axons of certain neurones – known as myelinated sheaths.) Think of fast motorways and slow bumpy country lanes.

Tissue irritation or injury initiates the release of chemicals (such as prostaglandins, histamine, peptides and kinins) that stimulate these nociceptors (like exhaust fumes being emitted from the car). When a receptor is stimulated, it causes the neurone to 'fire' (known as *cell depolarisation*) and an action potential of electrical energy conveys a message to a synapse. *Neurotransmitters* are the chemical messengers that cross this gap, for example, acetylcholine – with the neurone continuing to 'fire' along one of three established pain pathways (think of Postman Pat delivering his post in his van):

✔ **Dorsal Column Pathway:** Conveys information regarding where the pain response is occurring and vibration.

✔ **Spino-Thalamic Tract Pathway:** Conveys information of the pain site and the intensity.

✔ **Spino-Recticular Tract Pathway:** Involved within the limbic system, which is responsible for feelings and emotions.

These ascending pain pathways therefore stimulate areas of the brain and explain the subjectivity of pain perception: it's due to the incorporation of physiological, social and psychological elements, which is why anxiety often makes the pain experience worse.

Pain perception is a complex process, which Melzack and Wall attempted to explain with the development of the 'Gate Control Theory' in 1965. According to this theory, painful stimulus can be modified by a gating mechanism situated in the substantia gelantinosa in the dorsal horn of the spinal cord (grey matter that extends the whole length of the spinal cord and how the pain gets transmitted to the brain). The theory proposes that altering the transmission of pain is possible by deliberately activating another type of sensory receptor to dampen down the pain perception: for example, patients rubbing their arm after a subcutaneous injection. Rubbing the painful spot allows the rubbing signals to get through and block the pain signals. In other words, you can 'close the gate' or block the pain.

✔ Hot and cold applications

✔ Humour (as a coping mechanism)

✔ Keeping the patient informed about his condition (so he keeps 'control' of his condition)

✔ Listening to music

✔ Reducing anxiety and stress

✔ Relaxation therapies

Be aware of the saying 'each to her own': one method may not work for another patient. Personally, if you put on a Rod Stewart CD I'd be climbing the walls!

In this section, I take a look at a couple of ways of classifying and treating pain. For an idea of how the body experiences and communicates pain, read the nearby sidebar.

Classifying pain

To treat pain, you need to know what type of pain the patient is experiencing.

Pain can be classified according to how long it has lasted and what's happening in the nervous system. Many different types of pain exist – here are just four:

✔ **Acute pain:** In most cases, pain can be an acute, short-lasting event, such as a throb, dull ache or even a sharp, piercing soreness. Acute pain is accompanied by signs of hyperactivity in the autonomic nervous system, such as sweating and vasoconstriction. You can spot patients experiencing this type of pain by their body language, facial expressions and raised heart rate, even if they tell you that they're okay.

✔ **Chronic pain:** For some people, the pain can be long-lasting and may never go away. Chronic pain can severely affect your life, 'making every waking moment a misery' as one patient described it to me.

More specifically, chronic pain is often referred to as pain that lasts for more than six weeks (although some literature states a period of three months) and can be unbearable, making everyday activities difficult or impossible to manage. Chronic pain often produces changes in personality, lifestyle and activities of living.

Chronic pain is often more difficult to treat because it produces changes in the central nervous system (CNS), which causes changes in the autonomic nervous system – known as *adaption*. As a result, patients may not show many outward signs that they're in pain even though they are.

Don't fall into the trap of many inexperienced health carers, who can doubt that the pain even exists in the individual.

✔ **Neuropathic pain:** Doesn't require an external stimulus, but can be caused due to damage to the nervous system. Patients often describe it as 'electrical', 'tingling' or 'pins and needles'.

✔ **Nociceptive pain:** A response to an obvious stimulus, such as burning, cutting, broken bones and sprains, often described as 'deep', 'squeezing' and 'dull'. It may be accompanied by nausea and vomiting.

Climbing the analgesic ladder

The World Health Organisation devised the 'WHO Analgesic Ladder' to help health professionals manage a person's pain – tailored to the individual's needs. The ladder takes a stepped approach (see Figure 20-1) to the use of analgesics according to their 'group', as follows:

✔ **Simple analgesics:** Paracetamol and non-steroidal anti-inflammatory drugs (NSAIDs).

✔ **Weak opioids:** Tramadol, codeine.

✔ **Strong opioids:** Morphine, fentanyl, oxycodone, pethidine.

✔ **Adjuvants:** Drugs not originally devised for pain but found to be effective in difficult-to-manage pain. They include antidepressants and anticonvulsants.

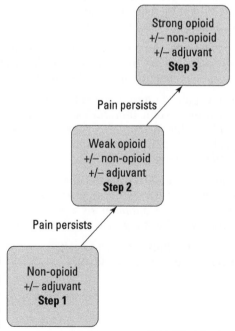

Figure 20-1: The analgesic ladder.

Opioids are drugs that bind to the opioid receptors within the central and peripheral nervous system and gastrointestinal tract. They're derived directly from the juice of the opium poppy. They include all the naturally occurring strong opiates, but also synthetic drugs with opiate-like or morphine-like qualities, for example, tramadol.

Heroin is known as *diamorphine* in healthcare settings.

Using (Not Abusing) Morphine

Intravenous (IV) morphine was traditionally administered in A&E and specialised clinical areas: theatre recovery, high dependency units, ICU and burns units. In contrast, wards usually administered oral or opiates via the intramuscular route.

Increasingly, however, IV morphine is being used in general wards (when acute pain is unmanageable with other analgesia and for patients just out of theatre), areas such as admission units, cardiology and so on, and where a change of dressing is required and the pain may not be managed with other analgesia.

Morphine works by inhibiting the release of chemicals from the dorsal horn fibres in the spinal cord, stopping the pain transmission: in other words, it silences the noxious impulses. Here's your guide to using morphine in the clinical setting.

Working out correct morphine dosages

Morphine can be administered by varying routes. The correct dosages for bolus morphine in the adult are as follows:

Route	Amount
Intramuscular (IM)	10 mg morphine IM hourly PRN (Pro re nata – as required)
Oral	10–20 mg oramorph 2-hourly PRN
Intravenous	Up to 10 mg in incremental doses (1–2 mg per dose – 1 mg for burn patients); 10 mg can be given in total, titrated according to the patient's condition

Titrating doses

In order to avoid over-sedation and/or respiratory depression, morphine must be titrated according to weight and age.

Knowing the predictors of dose

In adults, the main predictors are weight plus age. Special considerations apply for children who require IV morphine. The main predictor of dose is weight.

Administering morphine to elderly patients

Take extra care with patients over the age of 70 years old due to the following factors:

- ✔ Slower absorption
- ✔ Slower metabolism
- ✔ Slower excretory time
- ✔ Opiates being retained and so being effective for longer periods

You need to administer smaller doses (1 mg IV in incremental doses) and extend time between doses for equal effect without complications.

Ensuring balanced analgesia

You may wonder why patients having opiate medication require regular paracetamol and NSAIDs.

The answer is because paracetamol (acetaminophen) has what's called a *morphine sparing effect*, which means that it can 'pull out' the analgesic effect in order to reduce the total amount of morphine required to relieve the pain.

Non-steroidal anti-inflammatory drugs are useful adjuvants to the narcotic analgesia, because they can also enhance the activity of the narcotic, especially because they possess anti-inflammatory properties, helping to reduce any inflamed tissue.

Diluting IV morphine

The correct dilution for IV morphine is as follows:

1. **Add 10 mg morphine (1 ml) to 9 ml saline 0.9% in a 10-ml syringe, which equates to 10 ml of fluid in total in the syringe (each ml then contains 1 mg morphine).**

2. Administer 1–2 mg (2 ml) and wait for five minutes.

3. Monitor the effect (via pain assessment) and give a further 1–2 mg if necessary and repeat as necessary.

Being aware of complications and side effects

Always make patients aware of the potential complications/side effects of morphine:

- Constipation
- Hallucinations
- Nausea and vomiting
- Over-sedation
- Pain (headache and constipation)
- Pruritis (itching)
- Respiratory depression

Knowing the antidote to most opiates

If a patient has been given too much opiate, inform the doctor immediately. The general response in such situations is as follows:

1. Administer naloxone 400 micrograms per ml.

2. Dilute in 3 ml saline 0.9%, which equals 4 ml in total (each ml then contains 100 micrograms naloxone).

3. Administer in incremental doses of 100 micrograms (1 ml) and wait 2 minutes.

4. Repeat as necessary.

Assessing Patients and Documentation

As with all nursing care, you need to document accurately and robustly the things you do and don't do for your patients. You have to monitor those receiving opioid analgesia continually for the side effects I set out in the earlier 'Being aware of complications and side effects' section.

Performing observations

Observe patients continually during opiates administration. Perform observations every 15 minutes and for at least 30 minutes following the last dose of morphine.

Assessments include the following:

- ✔ Blood pressure and heart rate
- ✔ Nausea and vomiting
- ✔ Pain levels
- ✔ Respiratory rate and oxygen saturation
- ✔ Sedation levels

Completing the documentation

Clinical areas have assessment and observation charts. Pain observation charts usually have a sedation section.

Pay particular attention to the respiratory rate and sedation score. The purpose of administering opiate analgesia is to relieve the patient's pain, not to knock off his respiratory rate or comatose him.

Procedure for using acute pain assessment and observation chart

The acute pain assessment chart is designed to be used across all specialities, including patients with long-term chronic pain experiencing an acute exacerbation. This chart must be used for patients with acute pain, including those who receive opiates and all patients who've undergone surgery.

Perform normal observations of temperature, pulse rate and blood pressure as required; however, while doing these observations record the following information:

- ✔ **Respiratory rate:** During the time the patient is at rest, count the respiratory rate (for one minute) and record the data (as a number) in the line provided.

✔ **Sedation score:** Using the data below assess the patient, decide which of the following best matches and record the data (as a number) in the line provided:

- None: Awake and alert – 0
- Mild: Dozing intermittently – 1
- Moderate: Responds to painful stimulus – 2
- Severe: Difficult to rouse – 3

✔ **Pain score:** Question the patient: 'While you're resting, which of the following do you think best matches the pain you're experiencing?'

- No pain: 0
- Mild pain: 1
- Moderate pain: 2
- Severe pain: 3

Repeat the process: 'When you move, which of the following do you think best matches the pain you're experiencing?'

- No pain: 0
- Mild pain: 1
- Moderate pain: 2
- Severe pain: 3

Record the pain levels using a letter as follows: R = 'At rest'; M = 'Movement'; X = 'Both scores the same'

Record the data (as a number) in the grid provided.

✔ **Nausea score:** Assess the patient's nausea to evaluate the level of suffering at this time: None = O; Nausea = N; Vomiting = V.

Record the data (as a letter) in the line provided.

Monitoring and extra care for patients in main ward areas

Observe closely patients in general ward areas receiving opiate medication. The *syringe driver* – a machine to administer continuous medication, including morphine – is the preferred method of morphine administration on the main wards, together with the patient-controlled analgesia pump (PCA; see Chapter 14).

Undertake observations of the patient and machine at least hourly in main ward areas.

Syringe driver

The syringe driver (the general use of which I describe in Chapters 14 and 15) can deliver the medication in the syringe over a period of 1 to 24 hours. The medication, in this case the opiate, is drawn up into a syringe and mixed with an infusate, such as water for injection. The syringe is then attached to the syringe 'driver' or pump. The other end of the syringe has a line attached to a *cannula* (device going into patient's vein; see Chapter 16) into which the medication flows, in a controlled way.

You can administer the medication via a syringe driver into a patient via the following sites (among others):

- ✔ Anterior aspect of the upper arm
- ✔ Anterior chest wall
- ✔ Anterior aspect of the thighs
- ✔ Anterior abdominal wall

Each dose of IV morphine – whether a bolus or continuous infusion – is usually signed off by two members of appropriate staff (that is, two signatures required on the prescription chart).

Be aware of the person(s) you need to call if any problems arise.

Your patient is receiving IV morphine via a syringe driver and states that he feels nauseous. Is this a usual side effect to morphine?

Yes – common side effects are nausea and constipation. This patient should have an anti-emetic prescribed and administered. Also, this patient should have a softening and stimulating laxative (prophylaxis prescribed).

PCA pump

The PCA pump is a drug delivery system that patients control themselves, administering a prescribed amount of analgesia whenever they press a button. Pain has a psychological element, and so patient involvement and satisfaction can decrease anxiety and therefore reduce pain levels. For more details on PCA pumps, check out Chapter 14.

Part IV
Testing Your Calculations and IV Knowledge

Five ways to succeed at the test-yourself questions

- ✔ Discover where you stand with your healthcare-calculations knowledge.

- ✔ Identify any weak spots in your knowledge.

- ✔ Focus your revision efforts on the areas where you do less well in the test questions, including re-reading the relevant chapter.

- ✔ Practise writing out the commonly used formulae to increase your confidence.

- ✔ Remember that the more you practise, the more familiar the material becomes and the more your confidence grows.

web extras

Read the exclusive online article at http://www.dummies.com/extras/nursingcalculationsandivtherapyuk to help you know more about IV therapy.

In this part . . .

- ✔ Put the information you gain from this book into practice, to increase your understanding and knowledge.

- ✔ Test your IV therapy calculation skills.

- ✔ Revise for the calculations competence tests during your training.

- ✔ Prepare yourself for the IV calculations test prior to performing IV therapy for real.

Chapter 21

101 Questions to Test Your IV Therapy Knowledge

In This Chapter

▶ Trying out your IV therapy calculation skills

▶ Gaining confidence and competence with IV therapy

*W*hether you're reading this whole book, are just flicking through the sections you're interested in or haven't started it at all (because those DVD box sets are just too tempting), you may still want to assess how much you know about performing calculations and undertaking IV therapy correctly.

My aim with these questions is to give you confidence and competence in the clinical skill of IV therapy. So grab a pen and paper and get stuck in. If you don't have time to complete the 101 questions in one sitting, no problem – just dip in and out as time allows.

Don't worry if you're unsure how to approach a question – Chapter 22 gives you the answers and the relevant chapter in the book you may want to peruse.

1. IV digoxin comes as 500 micrograms in 2 ml. The prescription is to administer 400 micrograms of digoxin. What volume of digoxin do you administer?

2. Furosemide is available in a concentration of 20 mg in 2 ml. A patient is prescribed 10 mg IV as a bolus, to be given at a maximum rate of 4 mg/min:

    a) What volume of furosemide do you administer?

    b) Over how many minutes do you give it?

3. A patient has been receiving her heparin infusion through a pump, running at the following rates:

   - 1.4 ml for 6 hours

   - 1.2 ml for 6 hours

   - 1.1 ml for 6 hours

   - 1.3 ml for 6 hours

   What's the running total in 24 hours?

4. A doctor has prescribed one unit of blood for a patient. The blood is to run over 4 hours. The unit of blood consists of 350 ml. Calculate the drip rate in drops/min. The IV giving set (filtered) delivers 15 drops/ml.

5. An insulin infusion containing 50 units of human Actrapid has been diluted with 50 ml of sodium chloride, which has been running at:

   - 3 ml/hr for 3 hours

   - 3.5 ml/ hr for 2 hours

   - 2 ml/hr for 2 hours

   - 2.5 ml/hr for 1 hour

   - 4 ml/hr for 1 hour

   How many units of Actrapid insulin in total has the patient received?

6. Change 3,000 mg to grams.

7. Betamethasone valerate topical corticosteroid cream is presented as 0.1% w/w:

   a) What does w/w mean?

   b) How much active ingredient does this equate to in grams?

8. Round 0.1777777777777 to two decimal places.

9. How many tenths, hundredths and thousandths are in 0.962?

10. A patient has been prescribed one unit of blood. The blood is to run over three hours. The unit of blood consists of 415 ml. Calculate the drip rate in drops/min. The IV giving set (filtered) delivers 15 drops/ml.

11. A patient is prescribed 27 mg of Adenocor. Stock ampoules contain 30 mg in 10 ml. What volume of drug do you need to administer?

12. Work out the total input, total output and fluid balance for this patient:

    - Intake: IV fluid = 850 ml; oral fluid = 275 ml

    - Output: urine = 525 ml; vomit = 60 ml; wound drain = 50 ml

13. Change 0.95 grams to mg.

14. A child is prescribed 80 mg of paracetamol elixir. The drug is presented as 100 mg in 5 ml. Calculate the volume to administer.

15. 1 litre of Hartmann's solution is to be given over 12 hours. Using a volumetric pump, what's the flow rate?

16. What's $0.639 \times 1,000$?

17. Multiply 0.075 by 100.

18. Change 10 micrograms to mg.

19. Change 0.02 micrograms to nanograms.

20. What's considered to be the 'gold standard' cleaning agent?

21. Using the formula for working out body surface areas (BSA) and a calculator, what's the BSA for a small child weighing 18.2 kg and with a height of 110 cm?

22. What's a deficit of magnesium called? What are the normal serum levels for magnesium?

23. What's 'intracellular' space?

24. What's 51.4 divided by 1,000?

25. What are crystalloid intravenous fluids?

26. What does % v/v mean?

27. A patient's baseline APTT was recorded as 24 seconds. Six hours later his APTT is 31.2 seconds. Calculate the APTT ratio.

28. Anaphylaxis adrenalin ampoules contain 1 mg in 1 ml (1:1,000). What volume is needed for an IM injection of 500 micrograms?

29. Choose the least number of tablets for a 9 mg dose of diazepam (tablets are available in 2, 5 and 10 mg).

30. What's polypharmacy?

31. What are the World Health Organisation's '5 moments for hand hygiene'?

32. Dopamine is calculated as 120 mg/kg for a concentrated solution:

  a) Work out the dose for a baby weighing 1.4 kg.

  b) The pump is running at 0.25 ml/hr. How many micrograms/kg/minute is the baby receiving?

    Use the formula – amount in mg (answer from 32a) ÷ 50, ÷ weight × rate × 1,000 (convert to micrograms) and then ÷ 60 to get per minute = microgram/kg/minute.

33. Morphine 9 mg is needed and the stock solution is 15 mg in 1 ml. How much do you administer?

34. Diamorphine, made up to a total solution of 20 ml, is to be given over 24 hours using a syringe driver (pump). Calculate the rate in ml per hour.

35. Vancomycin comes as 500 mg in 10 ml. What volume do you draw up for a prescription of 400 mg?

36. In the world of blood, what's FFP?

37. Prescribed: 1 mg hydroxocobalamin IM injection. Stock: 1 mg/ml ampoules:

    a) How much of the drug do you administer?

    b) How is this injection to be given?

38. What's 3.49 correct to one decimal place?

39. Diamorphine hydrochloride 10 mg is to be reconstituted in 10 ml of water for injection. A patient is prescribed a 5 mg bolus intramuscular injection. What volume of the drug do you need to administer?

40. Amoxicillin is presented as 500 mg per ampoule. It's to be diluted to a volume of 10 ml. Your patient is prescribed 1.5 grams:

    a) What volume of amoxicillin do you draw up?

    b) The amoxicillin is to be added to a 50 ml bag of fluid and given at a rate of 2 mg/min. Over how many minutes do you give the infusion?

41. You need to infuse Aggrastat at 18 mg in 132 ml at 12 micrograms/kg/hr in a patient who weighs 14 kg. At what flow rate in ml/hr do you set the pump?

42. If you see a PR medication on a prescription chart, how do you administer it?

43. Solumedrol 2.5 mg/kg is ordered for a child weighing 15 kg: it's available as 125 mg/3 ml. How many ml do you administer?

44. A patient is prescribed 12.5 mg diazepam. Stock solution is 5 mg tablets. How many tablets do you administer?

45. Using the formula for finding the Body Mass Index (BMI) and a calculator, find the BMI for a woman with a height of 1.55 m and a weight of 120 kg.

46. Find the patient's Cardiac Output (CO) with the following readings:

    • Stroke volume: 75 ml

    • Pulse rate: 65 bpm

47. A patient is prescribed digoxin 125 micrograms. Stock is 0.25 mg. How many tablets do you administer?

48. What's a 'skin-tunnelled catheter'?

49. A baby weighing 0.9 kg is prescribed Vitamin K at 0.4 mg/kg IM. What dose should be administered and how?

50. Red blood cells are stored at what temperature in blood fridges?

51. Calculate the IV flow rate for 739 ml of 0.9% NaCL over 240 minutes IV in drops per minute.

52. What's a CVAD?

53. What are 'buffer' solutions?

54. Metoprolol tartrate (Lopressor) 18 g PO is ordered. Metoprolol is available as 18 g tablets. How many tablets do you need to administer?

55. Using the formula for working out body surface areas (BSA) and a calculator, what's the BSA for a small child weighing 14.5 kg and with a height of 95 cm?

56. Name the signs to alert you of hypovolaemia in patients.

57. Change 1.7 grams into mg.

58. If 2 ml of solution contains 5 mg of a drug, how much is in 8 ml?

59. Solumedrol 1.5 mg/kg is ordered for a child weighing 67 lb. It's available as 75 mg/1 ml. How many ml must you administer?

60. Work out the renal clearance of a patient with the following readings:

    - Urine: 50 mg/ml

    - Volume: 20 ml/min

    - Plasma: 40 mg/ml

61. What does w/v mean?

62. Using the formula for finding the Body Mass Index (BMI) and a calculator, find the BMI for a man with a height of 1.68 m and a weight of 70 kg.

63. Morphine dose is calculated as 2 mg/kg for a concentrated solution:

    a) A baby weighs 1.4 kg: how much morphine is prescribed?

    b) The pump is running at 0.5 ml/hr. How many micrograms/kg/hr is the baby receiving?

    Use the formula – amount in mg (your answer from 63a) ÷ 50 and then ÷ weight, × rate × 1,000 = micrograms/kg/hour.

64. Tablets are presented in combinations of 1, 2, 5 and 10 mg. What's the fewest number of tablets you can give for a prescription of 14 mg?

65. What's a deficit of sodium called? What's the normal serum level?

66. Name the six components of 'The Sepsis 6'.

67. Find the patient's Cardiac Output (CO) with the following readings:

  • Stroke volume: 65 ml

  • Pulse rate: 60 bpm

68. What's the most common trigger for anaphylaxis in children?

69. Is IV diazepam a Type A or Type B vesicant drug?

70. A patient is to receive 3 mg/1 ml of Adenocor, followed by a further 6 mg and then 12 mg, over a time span of six minutes. What volume does the patient receive in total?

71. Furosemide is available in a concentration of 20 mg in 2 ml. A patient is prescribed 30 mg intravenously as a bolus. This amount is to be given at a maximum rate of 4 mg/min:

  a) What volume of furosemide do you administer?

  b) Over how many minutes should it be given?

72. What's a BUN blood test?

73. What observations need to be performed on patients receiving opiate medication?

74. 1,000 ml of fluid is dripping at 20 drops per minute. The IV set delivers 15 drops per millilitre. How long does the infusion take?

75. Heparin is dispensed as 5,000 units in 5 ml and 550 units have been prescribed. This amount is to be diluted to 48 ml with 0.9% sodium chloride and be given over 24 hours:

  a) What volume of heparin is required?

  b) How much dilutant is required?

  c) At what rate do you set the infusion pump?

76. What volume of pure Savlon do you need to prepare 1.5 litres of a 2% solution?

77. Flucloxacillin IV is prescribed for a baby at 50 mg/kg. The baby weighs 3.7 kg:

  a) How much is prescribed?

  b) It comes as 250 mg in 5 ml in water. How much do you give?

78. How much titrate enoxaparin (1.5 mg/kg) do you administer according to body weight to a patient who weighs 66 kg?

79. Give the definition of anaphylaxis.

80. You need to infuse Aggrastat at 12.5 mg in 290 ml at 11 micrograms/kg/hr in a patient who weighs 19 kg. At what flow rate in ml/hr do you set the pump?

81. Ampicillin 80 mg per kg per day is prescribed for a 90 kg man. You're to give the drug every six hours. Calculate a single dose.

82. What's a VIP assessment?

83. Divide 20 in the ratio of 3:2.

84. LASIX 8,000,000 micrograms IV bolus is ordered. The drug is available 9 g in 5 ml. How much do you draw up?

85. When peripherally cannulating, what are six ways of encouraging the veins to dilate?

86. What are the symptoms of hypernatraemia in individuals?

87. Clear IV fluids use an administration set delivering how many drops per ml?

88. What's the normal value of urine specific gravity (SG)?

89. What does a high urine SG indicate?

90. Work out the forcibly exhaled volume (FEV_1) of this patient: FEV of 4.5 litres and a forced vital capacity (FVC) of 5.2 litres.

91. Change 3.21 to a whole number.

92. What's the antidote to most opiates?

93. What's a PICC, as in PICC line?

94. Work out the renal clearance of a patient with the following readings:

    - Urine: 70 mg/ml
    - Volume: 120 ml/min
    - Plasma: 50 mg/ml

95. When performing a neurological assessment, what's AVPU?

96. What volume of digoxin do you give to a patient in the following situation:

    - What you want = 275 micrograms
    - What you've got = 500 micrograms/2 ml

97. A patient is to have 2 litres of clear fluid in 24 hours. She has received 1,500 ml in 6 hours. How many drops per minute are required to correct the infusion?

98. Reconstitute the 500 mg amoxicillin sodium to make a total amount of 10 ml with water for injection (WFI). Displacement value = 250 mg/0.25 ml. An elderly patient is prescribed 250 mg to be given at a maximum rate of 2 mg/min.

a) How many ml of WFI do you add to the vial?

b) What volume of the drug do you draw up and administer?

c) Over how many minutes do you give the drug?

99. Heparin is presented as 20,000 in 20 ml:

a) How many units are present in 1 ml?

b) The patient weighs 82 kg. Calculate how many units the patient requires (18 units/kg/hr).

c) Chart states 80–89 kg = 1.4 (1,400 units) per hour. The APTT rate was recorded after 6 hours. Previously the patient was receiving 1.4 ml per hour according to her weight. The APTT is 2.52, which means that the rate must be reduced by 0.1 ml (100 units) per hour.

What's the new pump rate?

Note: If APTT is less than 1.2 or greater than 4, inform medical staff and document action in medical notes.

100. A patient is to be given 1 litre of sodium chloride 0.9% over six hours. Calculate the drip rate in drops/min. The IV set delivers 20 drops/ml.

101. A child is to receive 20 mg of pethidine, presented as 50 mg in 1 ml. What volume do you draw up?

Chapter 22

101 Answers to the IV Therapy Questions

. . . .

In This Chapter

▶ Checking out your IV therapy knowledge

▶ Moving confidently into the IV world

. . . .

When you've had a go at the questions in Chapter 21, see how you did with all these answers! Even if some of your answers to the drugs questions aren't the dosages that you're used to administering, remember that the point is more about whether your answer to the specific question is correct.

If you're ever in doubt when administering IV therapy, always check your answers to your calculations with colleagues, the British National Formulary (current addition), pharmacists or doctors.

Question	Answer	Chapter
1. IV digoxin comes as 500 micrograms in 2 ml. The prescription is to administer 400 micrograms of digoxin. What volume of digoxin do you administer?	Use this formula: What you want/What you've got × Volume 400 micrograms/500 micrograms × 2 ml = 1.6 ml	Chapter 8
2. Furosemide is available in a concentration of 20 mg in 2 ml. A patient is prescribed 10 mg IV as a bolus, to be given at a maximum rate of 4 mg/min: a) What volume of furosemide do you administer? b) Over how many minutes do you give it?	(a) Use this formula: What you want/What you've got × Volume 10 mg/20 mg × 2 ml = 1 ml (b) Use this formula: Dose prescribed/Rate 10 mg/4 mg/min = 2.5 = 2½ minutes	Chapters 8 and 14

(continued)

(continued)

Question	Answer	Chapter
3. A patient has been receiving her heparin infusion through a pump, running at the following rates: • 1.4 ml for 6 hours • 1.2 ml for 6 hours • 1.1 ml for 6 hours • 1.3 ml for 6 hours What's the running total in 24 hours?	$1.4 \times 6 = 8.4$ $1.2 \times 6 = 7.2$ $1.1 \times 6 = 6.6$ $1.3 \times 6 = 7.8 = 30$ ml *Note:* If APTT is less than 1.2 or greater than 4, inform medical staff and document action in medical notes.	Chapter 8
4. A doctor has prescribed one unit of blood for a patient. The blood is to run over 4 hours. The unit of blood consists of 350 ml. Calculate the drip rate in drops/min. The IV giving set (filtered) delivers 15 drops/ml.	Use this formula: Volume in ml/Time in hours × Drops per ml/ 60 min per hour $350/4 \times 15/60 = 21.87 = 22$ drops per minute	Chapter 14
5. An insulin infusion containing 50 units of human Actrapid has been diluted with 50 ml of sodium chloride, which has been running at: • 3 ml/hr for 3 hours • 3.5 ml/ hr for 2 hours • 2 ml/hr for 2 hours • 2.5 ml/hr for 1 hour • 4 ml/hr for 1 hour How many units of Actrapid insulin in total has the patient received?	3 ml/hr $\times 3$ hours $= 9.0$ ml 3.5 ml/hr $\times 2$ hours $= 7.0$ ml 2 ml/hr $\times 2$ hours $= 4.0$ ml 2.5 ml/hr $\times 1$ hour $= 2.5$ ml 4 ml/hr $\times 1$ hour $= 4.0$ ml 26.5 units of Actrapid have been received.	Chapter 8
6. Change 3,000 mg to grams.	3,000 mg divided by 1,000 = 3 grams	Chapter 2

Question	Answer	Chapter
7. Betamethasone valerate topical corticosteroid cream is presented as 0.1% w/w: a) What does w/w mean? b) How much active ingredient does this equate to in grams?	(a) weight in weight (b) 0.1 grams of betamethasone balerate in 100 grams	Chapter 5
8. Round 0.1777777777777 to two decimal places.	0.18	Chapter 3
9. How many tenths, hundredths and thousandths are in 0.962?	9 tenths; 6 hundredths; 2 thousandths	Chapter 2
10. A patient has been prescribed one unit of blood. The blood is to run over 3 hours. The unit of blood consists of 415 ml. Calculate the drip rate in drops/min. The IV giving set (filtered) delivers 15 drops/ml.	Use this formula: Volume/time × Drops per ml/60 min 415/3 × 15/60 = 34.58 = 35 drops/min	Chapter 14
11. A patient is prescribed 27 mg of Adenocor. Stock ampoules contain 30 mg in 10 ml. What volume of drug do you need to administer?	Use this formula: What you want/What you've got × Volume 27 mg/30 mg × 10 ml = 9 ml	Chapter 8
12. Work out the total input, total output and fluid balance for this patient: • Intake: IV fluid = 850 ml; oral fluid = 275 ml • Output: urine = 525 ml; vomit = 60 ml; wound drain = 50 ml	Fluid balance 1,125 − 635 = 490 ml	Chapter 7
13. Change 0.95 grams to mg.	0.95 grams × 1,000 = 950 mg	Chapter 2
14. A child is prescribed 80 mg of paracetamol elixir. The drug is presented as 100 mg in 5 ml. Calculate the volume to administer.	Use this formula: What you want/What you've got × Volume 80 mg/100 mg × 5 ml = 4 ml	Chapter 8

(continued)

(continued)

Question	Answer	Chapter
15. 1 litre of Hartmann's solution is to be given over 12 hours. Using a volumetric pump, what's the flow rate?	Use this formula: Volume/Time 1,000 ml/12 = 83.33 ml/hour	Chapter 14
16. What's $0.639 \times 1,000$?	639	Chapter 2
17. Multiply 0.075 by 100.	7.5	Chapter 2
18. Change 10 micrograms to mg.	10 micrograms divided by 1,000 = 0.01 mg	Chapter 2
19. Change 0.02 micrograms to nanograms.	0.02 micrograms multiplied by 1,000 = 20 nanograms	Chapter 2
20. What's considered to be the 'gold standard' cleaning agent?	Liquid soap, because bars of soap, in a communal place, contain skin cells and so on from previous users so pose an infection risk.	Chapter 18
21. Using the formula for working out body surface areas (BSA) and a calculator, what's the BSA for a small child weighing 18.2 kg and a height of 110 cm?	Use this formula: $(\text{Weight} \times \text{Height})/3{,}600$ $(110 \times 18.2)/3{,}600$ Step 1: $110 \times 18.2 = 2{,}002$ Step 2: Divide 2,002 by 3,600 = 0.556 Step 3: Find the square root of $0.556 = 0.745 \text{ m}^2$	Chapter 12
22. What's a deficit of magnesium called? What are the normal serum levels for magnesium?	Hypomagnesaemia Normal serum levels: 0.7–1.0 mmol/l	Chapter 15
23. What's 'intracellular' space?	The space within all body cells	Chapter 14
24. What's 51.4 divided by 1,000?	0.0514	Chapter 2

Question	Answer	Chapter
25. What are crystalloid intravenous fluids?	Aqueous solutions of mineral salts or other water-soluble molecules, meaning that they dissolve in water and contain electrolytes. Crystalloids tend to create low osmotic pressure, allowing fluids to move across the blood vessels, which can be linked to oedema. They tend to be much cheaper than colloids (blood, albumin, plasma and so on). Crystalloids are categorised according to their osmolarity compared with PLASMA osmolarity.	Chapter 14
26. What does % v/v mean?	Volume in volume = Number of ml in 100 ml	Chapter 5
27. A patient's baseline APTT was recorded as 24 seconds. Six hours later his APTT is 31.2 seconds. Calculate the APTT ratio.	31.2 seconds/24 seconds = 1.3 seconds	Chapter 15
28. Anaphylaxis adrenaline ampoules contain 1 mg in 1 ml (1:1,000). What volume is needed for an IM injection of 500 micrograms?	Use this formula: What you want/What you've got $\times$ Volume First change 500 micrograms into mg (500 divided by 1,000). 0.5 mg/1.0 mg $\times$ 1 ml = 0.5 ml	Chapter 8
29. Choose the least number of tablets for a 9 mg dose of diazepam (tablets are available in 2, 5 and 10 mg).	5 mg + 2 mg + 2 mg = 3 tablets	Chapter 8
30. What's polypharmacy?	When an individual takes four or more medications per day.	Chapter 14

(continued)

(continued)

Question	Answer	Chapter
31. What are the World Health Organisation's '5 moments for hand hygiene'?	Before touching a patient Before clean/aseptic procedures are to be used After body fluid exposure/risk After touching a patient After touching a person's surroundings	Chapter 18
32. Dopamine is calculated as 120 mg/kg for a concentrated solution: a) Work out the dose for a baby weighing 1.4 kg. b) The pump is running at 0.25 ml/hr. How many micrograms/kg/minute is the baby receiving? Use the formula – amount in mg (answer from 32a) ÷ 50, ÷ weight × rate × 1,000 (convert to micrograms) and then ÷ 60 to get per minute = microgram/kg/minute.	Use this formula: Weight (kg) × Dose a) 1.4 kg × 120 mg/kg = 168 mg b) 168 mg/50/1.4 kg × 0.25 ml/hr × 1,000/60 = 10 micrograms/kg/min	Chapter 8
33. Morphine 9 mg is needed and the stock solution is 15 mg in 1 ml. How much do you administer?	Use this formula: What you want/What you've got × Volume 9 mg/15 mg × 1 ml = 0.6 ml	Chapter 8
34. Diamorphine, made up to a total solution of 20 ml, is to be given over 24 hours using a syringe driver (pump). Calculate the rate in ml per hour.	Use this formula: Volume/Time 20 ml/24 = 0.83 ml/hour	Chapter 14
35. Vancomycin comes as 500 mg in 10 ml. What volume do you draw up for a prescription of 400 mg?	400 mg/500 mg × 10 ml = 8 ml	Chapter 8

Question	Answer	Chapter
36. In the world of blood, what's FFP?	Fresh frozen plasma	Chapter 17
37. Prescribed: 1 mg hydroxo-cobalamin IM injection. Stock: 1 mg/ml ampoules:	Drug = 1 mg per 1 ml. Therefore, to administer 1 mg = 1 ml. Using the formula:	Chapters 8 and 10
a) How much of the drug do you administer?	$1 \text{ mg}/1 \text{ mg} \times 1 \text{ ml}$	
b) How is this injection to be given?	By intramuscular injection	
38. What's 3.49 correct to one decimal place?	The rule is: if the second decimal place is 5 or more, add one to the first decimal place; if the second decimal place is less than 5, leave the first decimal place as it is.	Chapter 5
	In this case, 3.49 = 3.5	
39. Diamorphine hydrochloride 10 mg is to be reconstituted in 10 ml of water for injection. A patient is prescribed a 5 mg bolus intra-muscular injection. What volume of the drug do you need to administer?	Use this formula: What you want/What you've got $\times$ Volume $5 \text{ mg}/10 \text{ mg} \times 10 \text{ ml} = 5 \text{ ml}$	Chapter 8
40. Amoxicillin is presented as 500 mg per ampoule. It's to be diluted to a volume of 10 ml. Your patient is prescribed 1.5 grams:	Use these formulae: What you want/What you've got $\times$ Volume a) $1{,}500/500 \times 10 = 30$ ml	Chapters 8 and 14
a) What volume of amoxicillin do you draw up?	(***Note:*** 1.5 grams = 1,500 mg)	
	b) Dose prescribed/Rate	
b) The amoxicillin is to be added to a 50 ml bag of fluid and given at a rate of 2 mg/min. Over how many minutes do you give the infusion?	$1{,}500/2 \text{ mg/min} = 750 \text{ min}$ ***Note:*** Question asks for answer in minutes, not hours = 12 and a half hours	

(continued)

(continued)

Question	Answer	Chapter
41. You need to infuse Aggrastat at 18 mg in 132 ml at 12 micrograms/kg/hr in a patient who weighs 14 kg. At what flow rate in ml/hr do you set the pump?	Weight (kg) × Dose 14 kg × 12 micrograms = 168 micrograms Change 168 micrograms into mg = 168/1,000 = 0.168 mg Then use: What you want/What you've got × Volume 0.168 mg/18 mg × 132 ml/hr = 1.23 ml/hr	Chapters 8 and 14
42. If you see a PR medication on a prescription chart, how do you administer it?	Per Rectum = rectally	Chapter 6
43. Solumedrol 2.5 mg/kg is ordered for a child weighing 15 kg: it's available as 125 mg/3 ml. How many ml do you administer?	Use these formulae: Weight (kg) × Dose 15 kg × 2.5 mg = 37.5 mg What you want/What you've got × Volume 37.5 mg/125 mg × 3 ml = 0.9 ml	Chapters 7 and 14
44. A patient is prescribed 12.5 mg diazepam. Stock solution is 5 mg tablets. How many tablets do you administer?	Use this formula: What you want/What you've got 12.5 mg/5 mg = 2½ tablets	Chapter 8
45. Using the formula for finding the Body Mass Index (BMI) and a calculator, find the BMI for a woman with a height of 1.55 m and a weight of 120 kg.	Step 1: Height squared = 1.55 × 1.55 = 2.40 Step 2: 120/2.40 = 50.0 BMI (Obesity Class III – Very Severe)	Chapter 12
46. Find the patient's Cardiac Output (CO) with the following readings: • Stroke volume: 75 ml • Pulse rate: 65 bpm	Cardiac Output = Stroke Volume × beats per min (pulse rate) or SV × P = ml/min: 75 × 65 = 4875 ml/min	Chapter 12

Question	Answer	Chapter
47. A patient is prescribed digoxin 125 micrograms. Stock is 0.25 mg. How many tablets do you administer?	First change 125 micrograms into mg: 125 micrograms ÷ 1,000 = 0.125 mg Then use: What you want/What you've got 0.125/0.25 = ½ tablet	Chapter 7
48. What's a 'skin-tunnelled catheter'?	Long-term device that lies in a subcutaneous tunnel (between the sternum and the nipple) in order to enter a central vein – usually subclavian, or jugular, axillary or femoral, with the tip of the line usually placed at the superior vena cava junction. These devices are used if peripheral vascular access is problematic.	Chapter 16
49. A baby weighing 0.9 kg is prescribed Vitamin K at 0.4 mg/kg IM. What dose should be administered and how?	Use this formula: Weight (kg) × Dose 0.9 kg × 0.4 mg = 0.36 mg (IM = intramuscularly) You would then need to know how many mls to administer, after you know how the drug is prescribed.	Chapters 8 and 6
50. Red blood cells are stored at what temperature in blood fridges?	2–6 degrees Celsius.	Chapter 17
51. Calculate the IV flow rate for 739 ml of 0.9% NaCL over 240 minutes IV in drops per minute.	Change 240 minutes into hours = 240 min/ 60 = 4 hours Use this formula: Volume/Time (hours) × Drops per ml/60 min 739/4 × 20/60 = 61.58 drops/min = 62 drops/min	Chapter 14
52. What's a CVAD?	A central venous access device	Chapter 16
53. What are 'buffer' solutions?	Solutions used to correct acidosis or alkalosis. Lactated Ringer's solution has some buffering effect, but the main buffering solution is intravenous sodium bicarbonate.	Chapter 14

(continued)

(continued)

Question	Answer	Chapter
54. Metoprolol tartrate (Lopressor) 18 g PO is ordered. Metoprolol is available as 18 g tablets. How many tablets do you need to administer?	Use this formula: What you want/What you've got 18 g/18 g = 1 tablet	Chapter 8
55. Using the formula for working out body surface areas (BSA) and a calculator, what's the BSA for a small child weighing 14.5 kg and a height of 95 cm?	Use this formula: $(Weight \times Height) \times 3,600$ $(95 \times 14.5) \times 3,600$ Step 1: $95 \times 14.5 = 1377.5$ Step 2: Divide 1,377.5 by 3,600 = 0.382 Step 3: Find the square root of $0.382 = 0.618 \text{ m}^2$	Chapter 8
56. Name the signs to alert you of hypovolaemia in patients.	Thirst Acute weight loss Decreased skin *turgor* (ability of the skin to return to its normal shape when gently pinched) Clammy skin Decreased urine output *(oliguria)* Dark, concentrated urine A weak rapid pulse Altered mental status Flattened jugular veins when lying down Hypotension in usually normotensive patients Decreased central venous pressure	Chapter 15
57. Change 1.7 grams into mg.	$1.7 \times 1,000 = 1,700 \text{ mg}$	Chapter 2
58. If 2 ml of solution contains 5 mg of a drug, how much is in 8 ml?	$2 \text{ ml} \times 4 = 8 \text{ ml}$ $5 \text{ mg} \times 4 = 20 \text{ mg}$	Chapter 8

Question	Answer	Chapter
59. Solumedrol 1.5 mg/kg is ordered for a child weighing 67 lb. It's available as 75 mg/1 ml. How many ml must you administer?	Convert lb to kg (divide by 2.2): 67/2.2 = 30.45 kg Use these formulae: Weight (kg) × Dose 30.45 × 1.5 = 45.675 mg What you want/What you've got × Volume 45.675 mg/75 mg × 1 = 0.609 ml = 0.61 ml	Chapter 8
60. Work out the renal clearance of a patient with the following readings: • Urine: 50 mg/ml • Volume: 20 ml/min • Plasma: 40 mg/ml	Use this formula: Urine/Plasma × Volume 50/40 × 20 = 25 ml/min	Chapter 12
61. What does w/v mean?	Weight in volume. Number of grams in 100 ml.	Chapter 5
62. Using the formula for finding the Body Mass Index (BMI) and a calculator, find the BMI for a man with a height of 1.68 m and a weight of 70 kg.	Step 1: Height squared = 1.68 × 1.68 = 2.82 Step 2: 70/2.82 = 24.8 BMI (Normal)	Chapter 12
63. Morphine dose is calculated as 2 mg/kg for a concentrated solution: a) A baby weighs 1.4 kg: how much morphine is prescribed? b) The pump is running at 0.5 ml/hr. How many micrograms/kg/hr is the baby receiving? Use the formula – amount in mg (your answer from 63a) ÷ 50 and then ÷ weight, × rate × 1,000 = micrograms/kg/hour.	a) Weight (kg) × Dose 1.4 kg × 2 mg = 2.8 b) 2.8 mg/50/1.4 kg × 0.5 ml/hr × 1,000 = 20 micrograms/kg/hr	Chapter 12

(continued)

(continued)

Question	Answer	Chapter
64. Tablets are presented in combinations of 1, 2, 5 and 10 mg. What's the fewest number of tablets you can give for a prescription of 14 mg?	14 mg = 10 mg + 2 mg + 2 mg, therefore 3 tablets	Chapter 8
65. What's a deficit of sodium called? What's the normal serum level?	Hyponatraemia Normal serum levels: 133–146 mmol/l	Chapter 15
66. Name the six components of 'The Sepsis 6'.	1. Oxygen 2. IV Fluids 3. Blood cultures 4. IV antibiotics 5. Lactate and bloods 6. Urine output (fluid chart)	Chapter 18
67. Find the patients Cardiac Output (CO) with the following readings: • Stroke volume: 65 ml • Pulse rate: 60 bpm	Cardiac Output = Stroke Volume × beats per min (pulse rate) or SV × P = ml/min: $65 \times 60 = 3{,}900$ ml/min	Chapter 12
68. What's the most common trigger for anaphylaxis in children?	Food	Chapter 13
69. Is IV diazepam a Type A or Type B vesicant drug?	Type B	Chapter 19
70. A patient is to receive 3 mg/1 ml of Adenocor, followed by a further 6 mg and then 12 mg, over a time span of six minutes. What volume does the patient receive in total?	3 mg = 1 ml 6 mg = 2 ml 12 mg = 4 ml 21 mg = 7 ml	Chapter 8

Question	Answer	Chapter
71. Furosemide is available in a concentration of 20 mg in 2 ml. A patient is prescribed 30 mg intravenously as a bolus. This amount is to be given at a maximum rate of 4 mg/min: a) What volume of furosemide do you administer? b) Over how many minutes should it be given?	Use these formulae: a) What you want/What you've got × Volume 30/20 × 2 = 3 ml b) Dose prescribed/Rate 30/4 mg/min = 7.5 min	Chapters 8 and 14
72. What's a BUN blood test?	Blood urea nitrogen. A blood test to measure nitrogen in the blood, which comes from the waste product urea. Dehydration can raise BUN levels.	Chapter 19
73. What observations need to be performed on patients receiving opiate medication?	Patients receiving opiates have to be closely monitored, with patients continually being observed during administration. Observations need to be performed every 15 minutes and for at least 30 minutes following the last dose of morphine. Assessments include: Pain levels Sedation levels Respiratory rate and oxygen saturation Blood pressure and heart rate Incidence of nausea and vomiting	Chapter 20
74. 1,000 ml of fluid is dripping at 20 drops per minute. The IV set delivers 15 drops per millilitre. How long does the infusion take?	Use this formula: Vol/Rate × Drops per ml/min per hour 1,000/20 ×15/60 = 12.5 12 hours 30 min	Chapter 14

(continued)

(continued)

Question	Answer	Chapter
75. Heparin is dispensed as 5,000 units in 5 ml and 550 units have been prescribed. It's to be diluted to 48 ml with 0.9% sodium chloride and given over 24 hours: a) What volume of heparin is required? b) How much dilutant is required? c) At what rate do you set the infusion pump?	a) Use this formula: What you want/What you've got × Volume 550 units/5,000 units × 5 = 0.55 ml b) 50–0.55 ml = 47.45 ml dilutant c) Use this formula: Amount in syringe/Time 48/24 = 2 ml/hour	Chapters 8 and 15
76. What volume of pure Savlon do you need to prepare 1.5 litres of a 2% solution?	Use this formula: What you want/What you've got × Volume 2%/100% × 1,500 ml = 30 ml	Chapter 5
77. Flucloxacillin IV is prescribed for a baby at 50 mg/kg. The baby weighs 3.7 kg: a) How much is prescribed? b) It comes as 250 mg in 5 ml in water. How much do you give?	a) Use this formula: Weight (kg) × Dose 3.7 kg × 50 mg = 185 mg b) Use this formula: What you want/What you've got × Volume 185 mg/250 mg × 5 ml = 3.7 ml	Chapters 8 and 14
78. How much titrate enoxaparin (1.5 mg/kg) do you administer according to body weight to a patient who weighs 66 kg?	Use this formula: Dose × Weight 1.5 mg × 66 kg = 99 mg	Chapter 8
79. Give the definition of anaphylaxis.	A severe life-threatening generalised or systemic hypersensitivity reaction	Chapter 13

Question	Answer	Chapter
80. You need to infuse Aggrastat at 12.5 mg in 290 ml at 11 micrograms/kg/hr in a patient who weighs 19 kg. At what flow rate in ml/hr do you set the pump?	Use this formula: Weight (kg) × Dose 19 kg × 11 micrograms = 209 micrograms Change 209 micrograms into mg = 209/1,000 = 0.209 mg Use this formula: What you want/What you've got × Volume 0.209 mg/12.5 mg × 290 ml = 4.8488 = 4.85 ml/hr	Chapter 8
81. Ampicillin 80 mg per kg per day is prescribed for a 90 kg man. You're to give the drug every 6 hours. Calculate a single dose.	Use this formula: Dose per kg × Weight 80 × 90 = 7,200 mg (daily dose) Single dose (6 hourly) = 7,200/4 = 1,800 mg (or 1.8 grams)	Chapter 8
82. What's a VIP assessment?	Visual Infusion Phlebitis (a visual inspection of phlebitis)	Chapter 18
83. Divide 20 in the ratio of 3:2.	3 + 2 = 5, therefore 5 parts in total 5 parts = 20 and so one part = 20 ÷ 5 = 4 3 parts = 3 × 4 = 12 2 parts = 2 × 4 = 8 Ratio = 12:8	Chapter 4
84. LASIX 8,000,000 micrograms IV bolus is ordered. The drug is available 9 g in 5 ml. How much do you draw up?	Change micrograms into grams 8,000,000/1,000 = 8,000 mg 8,000 mg/1,000 = 8 g Use this formula: What you want/What you've got × Volume 8 g/9 g × 5 = 4.44 ml	Chapter 8

(continued)

(continued)

Question	Answer	Chapter
85. When peripherally can-nulating, what are six ways of encouraging the veins to dilate?	1. Using a tourniquet 2. Gravity 3. Opening and closing fist 4. Stroking the veins gently/lightly tapping 5. Applying heat 6. Applying a GTN patch	Chapter 16
86. What are the symptoms of hypernatraemia in individuals?	Observe for: *polydipsia* (excessive thirst), dry, sticky mucous mem-branes, flushed skin and elevated temperature in first instance. Agitation, mental status changes, seizures and coma.	Chapter 15
87. Clear IV fluids use an administration set delivering how many drops per ml?	20 drops/ml	Chapter 14
88. What's the normal value of urine specific gravity (SG)?	1.001–1.030	Chapter 19
89. What does a high urine SG indicate?	Dehydration	Chapter 19
90. Work out the forcibly exhaled volume (FEV_1) of this patient: FEV of 4.5 litres and a forced vital capacity (FVC) of 5.2 litres.	Use this formula: $FEV/FVC \times 100/1$ $4.5/5.2 \times 100/1 = 86.5\ FEV_1$	Chapter 12
91. Change 3.21 to a whole number.	If the number after the decimal point is 4 or less = round down. If the number after the decimal point is 5 or more, round up. 3.21 as whole number = 3	Chapter 3
92. What's the antidote to most opiates?	Nalaxone	Chapter 20
93. What's a PICC, as in PICC line?	Peripherally inserted central catheter	Chapter 16

Question	Answer	Chapter
94. Work out the renal clearance of a patient with the following readings: • Urine: 70 mg/ml • Volume: 120 ml/min • Plasma: 50 mg/ml	Use this formula: Urine/Plasma × Volume 70/50× 120 = 168 ml/min	Chapter 12
95. When performing a neu-rological assessment, what's AVPU?	Neurological response: A = Alert V = Verbal P = Pain U = Unresponsive	Chapter 7
96. What volume of digoxin do you give to a patient in the fol-lowing situation: • What you want = 275 micrograms • What you've got = 500 micrograms/2 ml	275 micrograms/500 micrograms × 2 ml = 1.1 ml	Chapter 8
97. A patient is to have 2 litres of clear fluid in 24 hours. She has received 1,500 ml in 6 hours. How many drops per minute are required to correct the infusion?	Fluid left to infuse: 2,000 ml – 1500 = 500 ml Hours left to infuse: 24 – 6 = 18 hours Use this formula: Vol/Time in hours × Drops per ml/min per hour 500/18 × 20/60 = 9.25 = 10 drops/min (9 if using the rule of 5s, but usually tend to round up with drip rates drops)	Chapter 14

(continued)

(continued)

Question	Answer	Chapter
98. Reconstitute the 500 mg amoxicillin sodium to make a total amount of 10 ml with water for injection (WFI). Displacement value = 250 mg/0.25 ml. An elderly patient is prescribed 250 mg to be given at a maximum rate of 2 mg/min. a) How many ml of WFI do you add to the vial? b) What volume of the drug do you draw up and administer? c) Over how many minutes do you give the drug?	a) 250 mg + 250 mg = 500 mg 0.25 ml + 0.25 ml = 0.5 ml 10 ml − 0.5 ml = 9.5 ml b) Use this formula: What you want/What you've got × Volume 250 mg/500 mg × 10 ml = 5 ml c) Use this formula: Dose prescribed/Rate 250 mg/2 mg/min = 125 min	(a) Chapter 14 (b and c) Chapter 8
99. Heparin is presented as 20,000 units in 20 ml: a) How many units are present in 1 ml? b) The patient weighs 82 kg. Calculate how many units the patient requires (18 units/kg/hr). c) Chart states 80–89 kg = 1.4 (1,400 units) per hour. The APTT rate was recorded after 6 hours. Previously the patient was receiving 1.4 ml per hour according to her weight. The APTT is 2.52, which means that the rate must be reduced by 0.1 ml (100 units) per hour. What's the new pump rate? **Note:** If APTT is less than 1.2 or greater than 4, inform medical staff and document action in medical notes.	a) 20,000 divided by 20 ml = 1,000 units b) Use this formula: Weight (kg) × Dose 82 kg × 18 units = 1476 units c) 1.4 ml − 0.1 ml = 1.3 ml	Chapters 7, 14 and 15

Question	Answer	Chapter
100. A patient is to be given 1 litre of sodium chloride 0.9% over 6 hours. Calculate the drip rate in drops/min. The IV set delivers 20 drops/ml.	Use this formula: Volume/Time in hours × Drops per ml/min per hour 1,000/6 × 20/60 = 55.5 = 56 drops/min	Chapter 14
101. A child is to receive 20 mg of pethidine, presented as 50 mg in 1 ml. What volume do you draw up?	Use this formula: What you want/What you've got × Volume 20 mg/50 mg × 1 ml = 0.4 ml	Chapter 8

Here's what your scores are telling you:

- ✔ **1–20:** Good try, though read sections of the book where you were wrong to increase your knowledge.

- ✔ **21–50:** Not bad, though re-read the sections for the question you got wrong.

- ✔ **51–80:** Very good, but don't get too cocky – just go over the sections you need to re-visit.

- ✔ **81–101:** Super professional status – share your skills with your colleagues and don't hide your intelligence under a bushel.

Part V
The Part of Tens

In this part . . .

- ✔ Work out the maths correctly to use the appropriate formula for the task in hand.

- ✔ Know the importance of using the aseptic technique to reduce the incidence of hospital-acquired infections.

- ✔ Understand the prescription chart abbreviations to minimise drug errors, such as not confusing milligrams (mg) with micrograms (mcg).

- ✔ Remember always to use the designated appropriate tools, such as the correct tourniquet, as opposed to improvising with what may be to hand: for example, examination gloves.

Chapter 23

Ten Tips for Administering IV Drugs Safely

In This Chapter

▶ Checking up on appropriate techniques

▶ Knowing the correct tools of the trade

*Y*ou never cut corners when administering IV drugs and fluids. You're only human (I assume; if you're not, note that aliens have a hard time becoming registered nurses!) and like all humans you can make mistakes. Therefore, in the world of IV therapy, you have to be extra vigilant to avoid harming your patients. No matter how busy, tired or cheesed off you are, you can never lose your ability to be kind and compassionate to patients, providing the best care you can at all times.

Here are ten important ways to keep your patients from harm when preparing IV drugs/fluids.

Employing the Aseptic Non-touch Technique

Shockingly, many patients die in UK hospitals every year from becoming infected after undergoing simple procedures, such as the insertion of a peripheral access device (cannula), due to poor hand hygiene and aseptic technique by the caregiver.

Using the aseptic non-touch technique (ANTT; see Chapter 1) is the key principle, where key parts of equipment, such as the cannula tip, aren't touched prior to insertion into the patient's vein, after you've followed the skin cleaning procedures I discuss in Chapter 18.

Also pay particular attention to the non-touch technique when preparing and administering IV medications (into central lines and so on) and drips. In short, wash your hands and always follow the ANTT principles.

Reading the Prescription

Take the time to become familiar with abbreviations on the prescription chart. Don't let prescribers fall into bad practice – for example, writing non-acceptable abbreviations on these charts, such as mcg or µg when they mean microgram (they need to write this term in full to avoid mistakes occurring).

Get to know drugs (generic and trade names) and their contra-indications, remembering at all times that your duty is to keep patients well, not make them sicker! Keep a copy of the most up-to-date British National Formulary close at hand to refer to and ask pharmacists and colleagues to assist you with any knowledge gaps.

Using the Correct Equipment

Being inventive and working with the tools you have at hand is great, such as using two 500-milligram ampoules of medication when you run out of the 1-gram ampoule. But sometimes, such inventiveness isn't good enough and you have to locate the correct equipment for the job.

For instance, if you have to administer packed red blood cells to a patient over three hours but have no pumps available in the clinical area, you don't administer this bag of blood by the gravity method of administration. Instead, you locate the correct piece of equipment (an IV volumetric pump) or ask a colleague to find one.

Some healthcare professionals still use gloves as tourniquets when undertaking venepuncture – but this practice is totally unacceptable. Only use gloves as part of the personal protection equipment. In short, use the equipment fit for purpose.

Choosing the Venous Access Device (VAD) Correctly

If a patient is critically ill, the usual practice is to insert the largest venous access device available (and often two of the devices).

In other cases, you need to make an assessment as to the most appropriate gauge size of cannula required. You take into consideration the patient's state of health and weight and the medication to be administered, as well as assessing the veins at the intended insertion site.

The golden rule is to use the smallest size cannula appropriate to the therapy into the largest available vein.

Working Out the Maths Correctly

In healthcare, you use mathematics constantly and your duty is to minimise drug administration errors. Initially, this responsibility is about remembering the decimal units and being able to convert one quantity into another. I give all the metric conversions in Chapter 2.

When you need to convert from micrograms to milligrams, you divide by 1,000 (because you're going up a size); when you need to convert milligrams to micrograms, you multiply by 1,000 (because you're going down a size).

Titrating Correctly According to the Patient's Body Weight

When medications need to be titrated according to the patient's body weight, you need to be able to convert decimal measures of weight from one unit to another (as I describe in Chapter 2), using the formula for working out the dose from Chapter 8: Weight (kg) × Dose.

The weight must be in kilograms when using this formula, and so you may need to make a conversion in some cases, using the information I provide in Chapter 2.

Delivering the Drug over a Set Time

Check for any timing considerations when administering medications. For instance, you have to inject certain medications over a given time period, such as those being given by bolus IV injection, so as not to cause speed shock (see Chapter 19). Speed shock is a sudden adverse physiological reaction to IV medication administered too quickly and can be caused by even tiny amounts of a drug.

Avoiding Coring of Rubber Bungs on Ampoules

When drawing up medications from ampoules with rubber bungs under the lid, ideally you want to use a specialised blunt filter needle. However, these needles aren't always readily available in all healthcare environments. Therefore, draw up the liquid with the smallest sized needle you can get away with to reduce the effect of drawing up particles of rubber from the receptacle (the same principle as for drawing up liquids from glass vials).

Insert the needle with the bevel side up, at an angle of 45–60 degrees. Before completing the insertion of the needle tip, lift the needle to a 90 degree angle to minimise the risk of the coring effect (see Chapter 19).

Reconstituting Drugs Correctly

Some drugs that are required to be freeze-dried or presented in powder format need to be reconstituted with liquid prior to administration – in other words, you take a drug and dissolve it in a solution.

When dissolved in the liquid, the powder takes up space in the receptacle. You need to take this into account when drawing up the total amount into the syringe, because the resulting solution has a greater volume than before – known as *displacement*. You need to take displacement values into account when dealing with small doses for neonates, or when drawing up partial ampoule or vial volumes. Check out Chapter 15 for how to calculate a dose using the displacement formula.

Priming the Lines

When patients require an IV drip, the administration line (or *giving set*) requires priming to expel the air. Otherwise, the patient receives a line full of air, before receiving the IV fluids, resulting in an air embolism (see Chapter 19).

When the drip chamber has been partially filled, open the flow regulator to allow the fluid to flush all the air from the tubing, taking care to use the ANTT (see the earlier section 'Employing the Aseptic Non-touch Technique'). In other words, you need to avoid contaminating the tip of the administration set until it has been attached to the access device.

Chapter 24

Ten Useful Drug-
Administration Formulae

*W*hen the patients are 'buzzing' for attention from their carers in the midst of the hustle and bustle of most clinical areas, you can sometimes have difficulty concentrating on working out your drug calculations to give medications safely.

Nevertheless, you can't let commotions distract you. If you have trouble remembering the correct formula – or maths and calculations aren't your bag (sorry, trying to be hip!) – never fear. This section gathers together ten formulae with easy-to-follow examples, all waiting to be picked (a bit like a singles bar for maths geeks). Go on, make friends with them now!

Working Out the Amount of Pills to Dispense

This formula is probably one of the most common you'll use:

What you want divided by What you've got

If your patient is prescribed 75 micrograms of thyroxine sodium and the tablets are available as 25-microgram ones, no problem: 75 divided by 25 = 3.

The patient requires three tablets – simple!

Calculating the Millilitres to Draw up for Liquid Medications

You use this ever-popular formula for injectables (like the expendables, only less wrinkly), including your bolus IV injections. It's also used for oral elixirs, syrups and emulsions. Remember that the answer is always in millilitres:

What you want divided by What you've got times Volume

Your patient is prescribed 125 micrograms of digoxin orally and digoxin is presented as 50 micrograms/millilitres. 125 micrograms divided by 50 micrograms multiplied by 1 millilitre = 2.5 millilitres.

Assessing Infusion Pump Rates

You call this formula (volume over the amount of time the fluids need to go through) into action in syringe driver pumps, in order to set the rate of the pump – for example, for insulin sliding scales. Confusingly, you also input these figures when administering IV bags of fluids – for example sodium chloride 0.9%, through a volumetric pump, and the pump works out the rate for you:

Amount of fluid (ml) divided by Infusion time (hours)

A doctor prescribes your patient 48 millilitres of fluid to be delivered over 24 hours: 48 divided by 24 hours = 2 ml/hour.

Of course, you use a different formula for the times your IV fluids are going through without a pump – using the gravity method (see the next two sections).

Computing IV Drip Rates – Gravity Method

This formula helps you to work out the drip rate in drops per minute when you're administering IV bags of fluid. The answer is in whole drops, because you can't count part of a drop (if you don't believe me, try it!).

The prescription states only the type and volume of fluid, leaving you to work out in which administration set you need to administer the fluid. Clear fluids such as sodium chloride 0.9% use an administration set delivering 20 drops per millilitre, whereas thickened fluids such as blood are administered in administration sets delivering 15 drops per millilitre:

> Volume in ml divided by Time in hours times Drops per ml divided by Minutes per hour

A patient is prescribed 1 litre of 'glucose 5%' to be given over eight hours. Using a standard administration set: 1,000 ml divided by 8, multiplied by 20 divided by 60 = 41.6 = 42 drops per minute (to the nearest whole drop).

Determining IV Drip Rates: Duration Request

You use this formula when administering a bag of IV fluids via the gravity method and you're asked how long the bag has left to run.

You first need to observe how much has been administered from the bag and how much is now left in the bag. You then put your amounts into the formulae, along with the rate that the bag was dripping (drops per minute):

> Volume in ml divided by Rate of infusion in drops per minute times drops per ml divided by Minutes per hour

A patient is receiving IV fluid hydration: 600 millilitres of fluid are left in the bag, which is dripping at 20 drops per minute, through an administration set delivering 15 drops per millilitre.

You're asked how long the infusion has left to take:

$600 \div 20 \times 15 \div 60 = 7.5 = 7\frac{1}{2}$ hours

Titrating Drugs According to Body Weight

In healthcare areas such as acute care, paediatrics or care of the elderly, many prescriptions rely on adjusting the amount according to the individual's body weight. The body weight part of this formula must be in kilograms:

Weight (kg) times Dose

A young child weighing 29 kilograms is prescribed '80 mg/kg/day' of a drug (in four doses per day): 29 multiplied by 80 = 2,320 milligrams of the drug per day divided by 4 = 580 milligrams per dose four times daily.

If it helps, you can reverse the wording to 'dose multiplied by weight'.

Administering an IV Dose per Minute

This formula works out over how long you need to administer your medications, such as IV bolus doses, in order to prevent speed shock (see Chapter 19):

Dose prescribed divided by Rate

Your patient is prescribed 20 milligrams of furosemide IV bolus. The correct amount has been drawn up and you need to administer this drug at a rate of 4 milligrams per minute: 20 mg divided by 4 mg = 5 minutes.

Counting Out Cardiac Output

This formula gives you the amount of blood pumped into the left ventricle in one minute. Severe infections can increase an individual's cardiac output, putting more pressure on the heart. The stroke volume (see Chapter 12) of the average person is between 60 and 80 ml of blood, in a standing position:

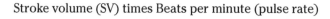

Stroke volume (SV) times Beats per minute (pulse rate)

A patient has a stroke volume of 65 millilitres with a pulse rate of 70 beats per minute: 65 multiplied by 70 = 4,550 ml/minute.

Measuring Body Surface Areas

When calculating drug dosages for neonates and children, using the body surface area (BSA; see Chapter 12) in square metres is more accurate than using the body weight formula. You work out the result and then find the square root of this resulting figure (using a calculator):

m^2 = square root of (height in cm × weight in kg) divided by 3,600

If you're asked to work out the BSA of a child weighing 15.2 kilograms whose height is 89 centimetres, here's the process:

1. **Multiply 89 by 15.2 divided by 3,600 = 0.375.**

2. **Find the square root of 0.375 (with a calculator) = 0.613 m^2.**

Filling up on Infant Feeding Requirements

With babies, you may need to work out their feeding volumes in order not to over- or underfeed them (Chapter 12 has more details). Infants should receive 150–200 millilitres per kilogram body weight per 24 hours:

Amount of milk (ml) times Weight of baby (kg) divided by Number of feeds in 24 hours

A baby weighing 4.5 kilograms requires six feeds per day:

✔ **Least amount:** 150 ml × 4.5 kg ÷ 6 = 112.5 ml

✔ **Most amount:** 200 ml × 4.5 kg ÷ 6 = 150 ml

Chapter 25

Ten Key Points When Administering Medication

In This Chapter

▷ Familiarising yourself with measurements and conversions

▷ Spotting adverse drug reactions

T
o keep your patients safe, follow these ten essential tips. Believe me, if you're ever admitted to hospital, you don't want to be treated by someone who doesn't follow them!

Taking Your Time

No matter what's going on around you, when administering medications to your patient, you need to focus on the task in hand. Many areas have dispensed with the traditional 'two to check' drug-administration rounds for routine medications, because the two nurses can get involved in conversation with each other and not concentrate fully on dispensing the medication.

Never rush drug administration. The golden rule is to take your time – less speed, more haste.

Knowing Your Abbreviations

Few abbreviations are permitted in the world of drug administration, but you need to know the ones that are used frequently.

Acquaint yourself with the acceptable abbreviations, such as IV (for intravenous), IM (for intramuscular injection) and PO (for 'by mouth') to name but a few. If you don't understand an abbreviation, ask someone!

Understanding Metric Measures and Calculations

Nurses have made mistakes and caused harm to people due to errors when converting between metric measures. Giving a patient 10 milligrams (mg) of a medication when the prescribed dose is 10 micrograms can have devastating consequences.

Always double-check your conversions and where the decimal point lies – for example, is the amount '10.0 mg' or '100.0 mg'?

When converting larger units to the next smaller unit, *multiply* by 1,000. When converting smaller units to the next larger unit, *divide* by 1,000.

Recognising Drugs that Look and Sound Alike

Many medicines have similar sounding names that you need to watch out for. Here are just a few: amoxycillin and ampicillin (broad spectrum penicillins); Ursogal (administered for the dissolution of gallstones) and Uftoral (given for the treatment of metastatic colorectal cancer); vinblastine, vindesine and vincristine (cancer medications).

Problems can also arise due to poorly written prescription charts, such as 'Does that say "Zantac" or "Xanax", I can't read the doctor's writing!' In this case, you must seek clarification.

Note that in this case, Zantac is prescribed for dyspepsia and benign gastric and duodenal ulcers, while Xanax (alprazolam) is prescribed for anxiety. The difficulty comes when you know that your patient suffers from dyspepsia and is highly anxious; the doctor may have prescribed either of these drugs!

Reviewing the Patient for Drug Allergies

Before administering any medication to patients, you must be aware of their allergy status. Even though the doctors have been through this issue with the patient, you also need to clarify that the person doesn't have an allergy to the drug you're administering. The problems come with drugs, such as piperacillin with tazobactam, which may not be easily recognisable as penicillin. The patient knows full well that she's allergic to penicillin, but unless you point out the nature of these drugs, she won't say so.

Being Aware of Adverse Drug Reactions and Contra-indications

Check the patient's medical history before administering medications. For example, a doctor may prescribe arachis oil to a patient in order to soften impacted faeces, but the patient has informed you that she's allergic to peanuts. Arachis is peanut oil so you shouldn't administer this medication and instead consult the doctor.

As a health professional you're not expected to follow the written prescription by the letter, but to look at the wider picture and communicate any concerns to the medical team.

Handling Sharps Carefully

No matter how busy you are, always clear away sharps immediately after use, to avoid needle-stick injuries to yourself, your colleagues, patients and visitors. Don't feel scared to tell doctors gently to remove their sharps if they start to walk away from them, whether these are injection needles or suture needles. Also, remember never to overfill a sharps bin. Check out Chapter 18 for more on sharps safety.

Asking for Advice and Information

No one expects you to know all the medications that patients can be prescribed. If you come up against a medication you've never heard about, your duty is to find out about it: indications, contra-indications, side effects and dose. The best starting place is the British National Formulary, plus pharmacy, patient information leaflets and colleagues.

Observing the 'Rights' of Medication Administration

Before administering medications, go through the mantra of the five 'rights' (or the ten if you prefer) from Chapter 6: right drug, patient, dose, route and time. Remember the items with this mnemonic: Don't let Patients Drink Raw Tuna.

Remembering Your Healthcare Responsibilities

You're responsible for your actions and omissions. For example, if a doctor prescribes lactulose constipation medication to a patient who already complained to you that morning that she'd been up all night with 'the runs', you'd document why you omitted the prescribed medication that morning.

Equally, if a patient was prescribed eptifibatide (a cardiac medication) for 10:00 a.m. that morning, and you forgot to administer it, this drug error is one for which you're answerable. Therefore, always check and recheck the prescription chart.

Index

• B •

• I •

• W •

• X •

• Y •

• Z •

About the Author

Claire Boyd has been in the nursing profession for 30 years, having the privilege of caring for a wide range of patients and their conditions. She started her nursing career as a support worker but always wanted to become a registered general nurse, so she obtained a place at university to undertake her nurse training. She has worked for the same NHS Trust since beginning her nursing career (seeing many changes over the years) before embarking on a Certificate of Education to become a practice development trainer, training nurses, doctors, assistant practitioners, operating department practitioners, support workers and student nurses in their clinical skills, including calculations and IV therapy.

She has written the Student Survival Skills series of books, including *Calculations Skills for Nurses, Clinical Skills for Nurses, Care Skills for Nurses, Medicine Management Skills for Nurses, Study Skills for Nurses* and *Communications Skills for Nurses,* all for John Wiley & Sons, Ltd.

She is also a holistic therapist, certificated in aromatherapy, massage and thermal-auricular therapy. Her colleagues and family enjoy her relaxation sessions, taking them to fragrant meadows, tropical islands and bubbling brooks – not literally but during these sessions!

Dedication

This book is dedicated to my wonderful husband Rob, my first love and soul mate. Thank you for everything you do for me, including taking all the photos in this book, and here's to the next 37 years of married life together!

I also dedicate this book to my children Simon and Louise, to my lovely son-in-law David, and to Owen – my first grandchild!

Author's Acknowledgments

Thanks go to the specialists in their field whom I pestered to get the information I required for the book – you know who you are. No person or animal was harmed while extracting this information!

Thanks also go to the great team at John Wiley & Sons, Ltd for their support and professionalism, namely Steve Edwards Chad Sievers, Andy Finch and Kim Vernon and to Miles Kendall for first approaching me to write this book.

Publisher's Acknowledgments

Executive Commissioning Editor: Annie Knight

Project Manager: Chad R. Sievers
and Steve Edwards

Development Editor: Andy Finch

Copy Editor: Kim Vernon

Technical Editor: Rosemary Lovell

Art Coordinator: Alicia B. South

Production Editor: Antony Sami

Cover Photos: ©iStock.com/milosluz